what to do
when you're having two

what to do
when you're having two

The Twins Survival Guide
from Pregnancy Through the First Year

NATALIE DIAZ

AVERY
a member of Penguin Group (USA)
New York

Published by the Penguin Group
Penguin Group (USA) LLC
375 Hudson Street
New York, New York 10014

USA · Canada · UK · Ireland · Australia
New Zealand · India · South Africa · China

penguin.com
A Penguin Random House Company

Most Avery books are available at special quantity discounts for bulk purchase for sales promotions, premiums,
fund-raising, and educational needs. Special books or book excerpts also can be created to fit specific needs.
For details, write: Special.Markets@us.penguingroup.com.

Library of Congress Cataloging-in-Publication Data

Diaz, Natalie.
What to do when you're having two: the twins survival guide from pregnancy
through the first year/Natalie Diaz.
p.   cm.
ISBN 978-1-58333-515-4
1. Twins.   2. Infants—Care.   3. Child rearing.   4. Multiple pregnancy.   I. Title.
HQ777.35 D53   2013   2013029177
306.875—dc23

Printed in the United States of America
3   5   7   9   10   8   6   4

BOOK DESIGN BY TANYA MAIBORODA

This book is dedicated to my sister,

Vivian Tracy Welsh.

You see things in me that only a big sister can.

You have been there since their very first breath

and have been my rock ever since.

I love you, sissy mouse.

contents

introduction

"THERE'S A HEARTBEAT," MY DOCTOR SAID DURING A SONOGRAM EIGHT weeks after my first in vitro fertilization (IVF). Apprehensive as I'd been that neither of the two embryos that had been implanted would take, I sighed with relief. Then a split second later he said, "And there's the second heartbeat," as if he had expected it.

I'll be honest. I definitely did not think, "Oh, this is wonderful." Instead, my gut reaction was, "I didn't sign up for this." Of course I knew that twins were a possible result of the IVF, but it had taken me so long to get pregnant that I hadn't seriously considered this. In that moment, I didn't know if I was happy or sad. I was in shock. I looked at my husband, John, for some sort of clue as to what I should be feeling. The first words out of his mouth were, "We'll have to move." I was overwhelmed, stunned, speechless, and frozen by the mere thought of the unexpected demands that we were about to face. Nothing could have prepared me for the impact that one moment would come to have on our entire lives.

Seven years later, I feel nostalgic about that time of intense anticipation. I look at Anna and John, our unbelievable twins, and I can laugh at all of the drama that came with bringing twins into the world and our trial-and-error attempts to efficiently care for them during their first year of life. It was frightening and challenging, but it was also crazy fun. Having twins can be scary, especially at first, but roller coasters are also scary, and those ups and downs are always thrilling.

Unless you come from a family with a history of twins, you are essentially on your own when it comes to knowing how to care for your twinnies. What works for a singleton, what parents of multiples refer to as a single birth child, may not prove useful for you. That goes for pregnancy, delivery, feeding the newborns, and beyond, so the advice that you get from your mother, aunts, sisters, and friends may not always apply. You have to either forge your own way or seek advice from those who have been there before you.

There are no other twins in my family, and after finding out that I was expecting a pair instead of one, I was desperate for information and a connection to other twin moms. At only fourteen panicked weeks pregnant, I attended my first Manhattan Twins Club meeting. Right away, I knew that the strangers in that room held the keys to my parenting success. They had been in the trenches and survived, and they had learned quite a bit in the process. They had the answers that I was looking for.

When we returned home after the drama of the premature birth and our babies' stay in the neonatal intensive care unit (NICU), I was so relieved to have those mentors who provided me with their hard-earned knowledge about how to handle two bundles of joy on three hours of sleep a night. I don't know what I would have done during that period of hormone-fueled slapstick as I attempted to care for and breast-feed those babies without the counsel of those wise women. I incorporated their recommendations, gained confidence, and learned my own tricks of the trade. Once my twins were thriving and I had successfully gotten through the newborn stage, I knew that I had to pass on my newfound wealth of experience. I became the director of the Manhattan Twins Club, served on the board of the New York State Mothers of Twins Club, and was the publicity coordinator for the National Organization of Mothers of Twins Clubs.

Most moms learn from their first child (or their first set of twins!) and then put that acquired wisdom to work on their subsequent children, but after my twins I wasn't able to have any more children. I needed my own outlet for all of my knowledge—something that would serve as my third "baby." As I saw how many women all over the country were in dire need of information about parenting twins (just as I had been), I decided to unite our community of twin parents with the launch of Twiniversity, an international online community exclusively for parents of multiples to exchange information, horror stories, advice, support, and friendship.

The motto of Twiniversity is, "Community, Knowledge, Humor," and that is exactly what you will find in this book. It is based on my own experience first and foremost, but also incorporates advice from other twin parents as well as experts in their fields, from financial advisers to ob-gyns. You'll get a realistic picture of what to expect during pregnancy and during your twins' first year, and receive endless tips on how to get through the day and streamline your life so you can enjoy those yummy babies to the maximum. Nothing is off-limits here, as we will delve into some pretty murky waters. Some of what you read on these pages may scare you, but rest assured I'll always give you a solution and tips that will get you through the hardest moments with a smile on your spit-up-covered face. Aren't you excited? Let's get started!

CHAPTER 1

make mine a double

I F YOU'RE ANYTHING LIKE ME, YOU MAY HAVE KNOWN THAT IT WAS possible for you to become pregnant with twins, either because you used some sort of reproductive technology to get pregnant (which increases the chances of having twins) or because twins run in your family. Many people don't realize that there is a gene for carrying fraternal twins. Some women are more likely to release more than one egg during a single ovulation cycle. So if your mother had a set of fraternal twins, you are more likely to do so, as well. Or maybe you got pregnant with twins spontaneously, have never even met a set of twins before, and just hit the jackpot! Either way, finding out that you're having twins definitely ranks among the most shocking moments of any parent's life. Somehow, even knowing that it's a possibility doesn't make it any more real. But hearing those two heartbeats makes it feel *really* real now, doesn't it?

Once you've come to terms with the concept of twins (or even before), your mind will probably start spinning with the thought of everything that you have to do in order to prepare yourself for these creatures' arrivals. This chapter will give you an overview, with checklists so that you know what you have to do, a pregnancy timeline so that you know exactly when you have to do it, and invaluable tips from me, the pros, and other twin parents so that you know the best way to get all this stuff done. But first, we'll talk about how to wrap your mind around the big news. Here we go.

Coming to Terms with Two

Be honest—what was your first thought when you found out that you were expecting twins? Were you shocked, terrified, overjoyed, or did you feel a combination of these emotions? Were you totally overwhelmed and confused about why you felt exactly the way you did? Even if you were trying to conceive for a long time or knew that twins were a possibility, it's quite likely that you felt a jumble of emotions when you learned the news. This is totally normal. Some people even have a very negative reaction. The truth is that the thought of having twins can be really scary.

You might start asking yourself questions like: How am I going to do this? How will I be able to carry them to term? Who is going to help me? Will I ever be able to go back to work? Will I ever get out of the house again? What's going to happen to my body? Are the babies going to be born healthy? Am I going to stay healthy? How are we going to be able to afford this?

If you've said any of these things to yourself, you are not alone. I think that shock is the first thing that any expectant mother feels when she learns that she is having twins, no matter how she got pregnant in the first place. As I already described, I was disappointed when I first learned that twins were in my future. Living in a tiny New York City apartment, a place that's not exactly accommodating to double strollers, I wondered how I could possibly fit twins into my lifestyle. Carrying and raising two babies at the same time was never on my radar. Heck, for years I couldn't even conceive. How could I have possibly imagined that I could conceive two babies?

Don't feel guilty if your immediate reaction to having twins also wasn't

> *From the MOM Squad:*   *"I was taken aback at first and just shocked, but as the days and weeks went on I have never felt more blessed and more privileged to be a mother of twins!"* —Brittanie W.

exactly to jump for joy. Parents in general can always find something to feel guilty about, and that goes double for parents of twins. I know this was true for me. Let it go. Decide right now that you refuse to feel guilty about anything because you're going to do your best and that's all you can do, anyway. You'll love those babies to the moon and back no matter what your initial reaction was to having twins. I can pretty much guarantee that. In the meantime, here are some tips that will help you mentally prepare for the reality that awaits you.

Get Support

Always remember that you have the support of other twin moms in your area and on the Twiniversity website twenty-four hours a day. Hearing the truth about what life with twins is like from moms who've been there may be sobering, but it will also be invaluable.

> *From the MOM Squad:*   *"Find a twin (or a moms of multiples) club as soon as possible. It was the best thing I've ever done. I made a lot of great friends that know exactly what I am going through and are able to help me through anything that happens."* —Sue Z.

Talk It Out

The best way to come to terms with this life-changing news is to talk about it. If you try to sweep it under the rug, it will eventually come back to bite you. I'm not saying that you have to immediately share it with the whole world (unless you want to), but it's important that you and your partner communicate openly so that you can both come to terms with the news together.

Take the Good with the Bad

Yes, this news is overwhelming. Yes, this news is scary. But guess what? This is going to be so much fun! My husband always describes having twins as the "best worst thing" that's ever happened to us, and that is completely accurate. When you hold those two babies in your arms for the very first time and look into their tiny little eyes and see yourself, you'll wonder why you ever worried about anything at all.

Focus on the Positive

A short list of the best parts of having twins

- You're basically growing someone along with their best friend. You won't ever have to worry about play dates and socialization, because your child's play date will always be right there.
- You'll only have to go through childbirth once for two kids.
- One of your twins will always want to snuggle. You'll get double the hugs and double the kisses!
- Three words: potty train once. (That's if you don't have any other children, of course.)
- You'll get the terrible twos for two kids over in one go.
- You'll never need to teach your children how to share. They will have shared you from the beginning, so they'll know exactly what sharing means.
- You'll also never have to teach them how to care for others. After getting to know hundreds of pairs of twins, I have found that twins are significantly more empathetic than the general population. Think about it—if you always had somebody right next to you who cried when you cried and you laughed when they laughed, you would basically have empathy built in, too.

Note from Dad: *"I spotted it before my wife or the sonogram tech did. They were both looking at where he was rubbing the wand on her belly. I was watching the monitor. As the tech wiggled it around, I saw two circles on the screen. I asked, 'Why are there two circles?' He stopped, turned around, and looked at the monitor. Then he turned back around and waved his wand around some more while looking at the screen. He said, 'I think you're right—you're having twins.' I couldn't even think at that point. I just leaned over and gave my wife a hug."* —Phil N.

My Two Dads (or Moms)

Many of our Twiniversity families are same-sex couples, and I hope you know how important you are to our community. We know that bringing twins into the world as a gay couple comes with its own unique challenges. Many gay dads who are expecting twins attend my classes. Because twins with gay fathers usually come into the world with the help of a traditional or gestational surrogate, there are special issues. One of the wonderful families I know says: "While on one hand neither you nor your partner is experiencing a difficult double pregnancy, a surrogate also puts you at a disadvantage. You won't experience a traditional transition to parenthood, so you'll need some extra help in preparing to become parents of two. Take parenting classes, read books, and hang out with parents and their children (preferably twins and/or infants). Ask them how they prepared and what parts of parenting twins they couldn't have prepared for. Offer to change diapers and feed the babies so that you get as much practice as possible. Make sure that you build a small, close-knit circle of support well before the birth. Join support groups for parents of twins and for gay parents. These can be virtual communities or groups that meet in person. Use your religious, school, work, and other affiliations to find people who may be in (or have experienced) a similar situation and are willing to meet and talk. Talk to your friends and family about your concerns and fears. Tell them how you want them to help. Actually ask them to help. For many, the experience of surrogacy radiates independence, and your community may get the feeling that you don't need any help, so make sure they know that you do.

"Many gay parents, especially dads, do not get the same parental leave that women get, which means that you may either need to take an unpaid leave of absence or pay for child care from the very beginning of your twins' lives. There is no magic solution for this except the general guidance of planning ahead and being creative.

"When your twins get older, you will want to tell them the story of how they arrived, so plan for this now by documenting the process in pictures, videos, anecdotes, and journal entries. Start collecting these pieces of written and visual media as soon as you can, and organize it so that when you want to put together a book, an album, or maybe a video, the information is there for you. Also think now about how you will respond to strangers' questions about where your twins came from—and know that you will receive many of these queries! Plan some simple stock answers that you feel comfortable with, like, 'We had these guys with the help of a surrogate,' so that you'll never get caught off guard. Whatever you choose to say, remember that being gay, out, and a parent is very brave. When you share your story with others, you are starting to tell your children the narrative of their birth, even if indirectly. Keep it coherent, and maintain the same level of integrity you would want to tell your children about how they came into the world."—Asaf R.

As for the mom/mom families in Twiniversity, we got a few bits of wisdom and advice from our member Laurie H., mom of eight-month-old twins. Laurie told us how being a two-mom family of twins actually made things easier. "I've known loads of two-mom families of singletons. Sometimes during infancy, both moms want to be maternal and hold and feed the baby. With twins we always have one, if not both, of them so who could be jealous?"

One of the challenges of being a two-mom family is often noticed when the moms have to carry the boys around in their car seats. "The physical element is often harder for us. We don't have a strong dad to carry the boys around, and as a result we always have our stroller." Laurie also explained how important it is to have the support of your community. "We are very lucky that we belong to CBST [Congregation Beit Simchat Torah in New York]; it's the city's LGBT synagogue. It's a great community with a true baby boom. This year there were eight sets of twins born; we were the only mom family!"

With same-sex marriages and births on the rise, Twiniversity has added a resource section exclusively for LGBT twin parents. Please visit www.Twiniversity.com when you get a chance for a list of great websites and research.

Doctor Dilemmas

Now that you're starting to become acclimated to the idea of twins, it's time to make sure that you know how to keep them (and you) healthy. Over the next year or so, you will probably see both your ob-gyn and your pediatrician more than your best friend, sister, or even your spouse, and so it is very important to choose someone who makes you feel comfortable and safe and whose office you won't dread visiting with every cell in your body. Many moms of twins assume that they just need to find a doctor who is experienced with twins, but there is more to it than that. Here is what you need to know about finding an ob-gyn and pediatrician for you and your twins.

Selecting an Obstetrician

When your pregnancy is first confirmed by a doctor, it will probably be your primary doctor, your gynecologist, or perhaps even a fertility specialist, but then what? Well, it's time to find a good obstetrician. How do you do that? A lot of this depends on where you live. First of all, you may have been planning to get pregnant and already found an OB you like. Congratulations! You can skip to the next section. Otherwise, here are my best tips for selecting your and your babies' first doctor.

GET A REFERRAL

You can make this very easy for yourself and have your current gynecologist make a referral for you, perhaps to someone else in her practice. This is not only convenient, but also saves a lot of time because they will already have your complete medical history in their files. If you find out that you need a high-risk doctor because of predetermined factors in your pregnancy (or perhaps discovered the need for a high-risk doc in past pregnancies), your gynecologist or obstetrician can help you choose one who is best for you.

What Is a High-Risk Obstetrician and Do You Need One?

It's not uncommon for an expectant parent of multiples to see a high-risk obstetrician, a specialist assigned to patients who have predetermined medical issues that might affect their pregnancy. It could be any condition, from a blood clotting disorder like the one I had to a heart problem. You may also need to see a high-risk obstetrician if complications develop during your pregnancy. At any time during your pregnancy, your obstetrician could refer you for an additional examination. If you do get a referral to see a high-risk doctor, don't set yourself into panic mode. Sometimes your doctor just wants to get a second opinion or may want to investigate a possible condition further but is limited by the sonogram equipment in her office. Don't worry until a doctor tells you to worry. Many parents of multiples visit both types of docs. Look on the bright side: you'll get more sonograms, which will give you more opportunities to see your babies.

CHECK YOUR INSURANCE

Most insurance companies require you to use a doctor in their network, and you can start by getting a list of approved obstetricians from them. Save yourself a ton of time by avoiding a situation where you carefully select a doctor and then discover too late that the medical practice doesn't accept your plan.

FACTOR IN LOCATION AND OFFICE HOURS

Don't assume that the most convenient doctor will be located close to your home. Depending on your schedule, it may make more sense to go to someone whose office is near your workplace. Think about your schedule and where you'll be around the time of most of your appointments. Consider office hours. When are you most likely to go to your appointments? Early in the morning before work, at lunchtime, or later in the evening? Make sure the doctor is accessible when you need her.

THINK ABOUT THE HOSPITAL WHERE YOU'LL DELIVER

It's time to consider where you plan to deliver these babies. If you have multiple hospitals in your area, you'll want to choose a doctor who has the right to deliver at the one you prefer. If you don't have a hospital preference (or choice), then choose the doctor you like best and go with his or her hospital affiliation.

MEET IN PERSON

Think about any other preferences that are important to you, like whether you want to see a male or a female doctor, and then make a list of the handful of doctors that you are interested in. Call their offices and see if you can schedule an initial meeting/interview. Here are a few questions to ask when you meet them:

- How many twins have you delivered?
- How many vaginal deliveries of twins have you performed?

- Do you treat parents of twins any differently than singleton moms—for example, by putting them on bed rest even if they don't have any symptoms? (Some doctors feel that any mother of twins should be off her feet after thirty weeks regardless of how she feels. This is a bit of an old-school philosophy, but some doctors still follow this practice and it is the kind of thing you'll want to find out during the interview process.)

Remember that most obstetricians work in a group practice, and the doctor delivering your babies will be the one in the practice who is on duty when you go into labor. In this case, make sure you meet all of the doctors in the practice so that you are comfortable with the person who shows up on the big day.

LISTEN TO YOUR GUT

Finally, you have to choose based on your comfort level. I'll tell you that the first obstetrician we saw during my pregnancy was not the doctor who delivered our twins. After our fertility specialist told us the good news, we asked for his referral. We quickly made an appointment with the doctor he referred us to, but after that first visit I knew that this doctor wasn't for us. Truthfully, I hated him, and I "hate" very few people in this world. In fact, I still carry a grudge, because he scared me into believing that I was going to deliver at twenty-seven weeks to twins with significant disabilities. I'm sure he meant well and just wanted to "prepare" me for things that might happen, but I can remember the trauma of that meeting like it was yesterday. We started searching around and found a terrific doctor who put us at ease.

Your to-do list may be a mile long, but take the time to interview obstetricians. You will be seeing this person once a month at first, and then weekly, and then perhaps daily as your delivery approaches. Make sure you like your doctor, feel comfortable with him or her, and share similar philosophies about pregnancy and childbirth. The person who delivers your twins will forever be part of your life story and theirs.

Having Twins via Surrogate?

Surrogacy is a wonderful way to bring babies into the world if you are unable to carry your own. But the process can be fraught with its own issues and unknowns. Having someone else carry your babies is very scary and overwhelming. You have to find peace and the ability to trust your surrogate. It is important to remind yourself that you selected this person because her body has an easier time carrying babies than yours. It may help to tell yourself, "She is good at this; being pregnant is easier for her."

During a surrogate pregnancy, don't forget to make this time special and to do things with your partner to prepare for the babies' arrival. Spend time preparing the nursery together and shopping for baby gear. Take a twins class, like the one offered by Twiniversity. (Hint, hint.) It probably took you a long time to reach this point, so you should enjoy it and experience the pregnancy in your own way. Don't shy away from baby showers or other celebrations that you feel comfortable with.

If you are considering a surrogate, you should know that there are many surrogacy options available both within the country and internationally. It is important to pick something that works for you and your partner. You may choose a surrogate who you talk to regularly and attend all doctors' appointments with in person or via video chat. Some people prefer to keep things more private and wish to receive medical updates via e-mail instead of forming a close, personal relationship with their surrogate. Others choose to stay in touch with their surrogate for years after the birth of their twins. These are all very personal decisions, and it is important to think about what feels right for you and your family.

Selecting a Pediatrician

What are your options for your twins' doctor? Preeti Parikh, MD, a board-certified pediatrician, explains:

"There are three main types of providers you can choose from for your children: A family medicine doctor, a nurse-practitioner, or a pediatrician.

Family medicine doctors must complete three years of residency after medical school. Family medicine residents train in pediatrics and several other areas such as internal medicine, orthopedics, and obstetrics and gynecology. They usually spend several months training in each area. Afterward, they're eligible to take the certifying examination of the American Board of Family Medicine.

"A pediatric nurse-practitioner (PNP) has earned a master's degree in nursing and can take medical histories, perform physical examinations on children, make medical diagnoses, write prescriptions, and provide counseling and treatment. PNPs may specialize in a particular area, such as neurology or endocrinology. PNPs work closely with doctors in hospitals, clinics, and private practices.

"And of course pediatricians are medical doctors who specialize in ages of newborns to young adults."

Once you decide what type of doctor you want for your twins, you should start looking for doctors between weeks twenty-four and thirty-four of your pregnancy. As always, the sooner you start the better. The first and most obvious tip is to ask around. Your local twins club is an excellent resource to find the top twinnie docs in your area. If you live in an area without a lot of options, you should definitely choose the pediatrician who is closest to your home. You will be visiting that doctor's office quite a bit in the coming years, so convenience is actually a really important factor. If you live in a town or city with numerous options, you should pick a few who have been recommended to you and interview them. Most doctors will be happy to meet with you before your twins' birth, and if one of the candidates on your list isn't willing to do so, then he or she just eliminated themselves. Thank them for saving your time!

Here are some good questions to ask during the pediatrician interview:
- Why did you become a pediatrician?
- Do you have a subspecialty or any special medical interests?
- How long have you been practicing medicine?

- Do you have any children? (Bonus points if they are a parent of multiples!)
- Are you authorized to work at the hospital where you are delivering?
- How much preemie experience do you have? (We'll talk more about this later.)
- What is your parenting philosophy on feeding (breast-feeding/bottle), sleep (cry it out, co-sleeping, etc.), and immunizations (bulk them/spread them out)?
- How much time do you allow for appointments?
- Will each child get his or her own appointment, or is it one per family?
- On average, how long is the wait in the waiting room?
- Do you have a separate waiting room for sick children? Do you put them right in the exam room?
- How can I contact you for nonemergency questions? E-mail? Text? Telephone?
- If I have to take the twins alone to the doctor, can you (or someone from the office) assist me?

Here are some things to think about after your interview with the doctor:

- How close is the office to your home? You'll be going to the pediatrician quite a lot for the next few years, so it really should be convenient.
- How long did you have to wait to ask your questions?
- Did you have a good feeling about the staff? Did they seem professional? Courteous? You'll be dealing with these people a lot on the phone and in person.
- How was the doctor's attitude toward the interview? You want to find someone who you feel comfortable talking to.

In addition to convenience/location, the most important thing is how you felt about the doctor and his or her office. No matter how experienced or brilliant a doctor may be, if this practitioner made you feel intimidated and uncomfortable asking your questions, rushed you through the visit, or communicated poorly, then this doctor may not be for you and your twins.

Insurance Information

Okay, now that you have your doctors squared away, it's time for a lesson on your insurance. Each insurer and each specific plan varies in terms of what is covered when it comes to pregnancy needs, baby gear, and the babies' medical needs. I'm not going to get involved in deciphering your medical bills, but I am going to give you a list of surprising things that your insurance company might cover. Call your carrier today and find out if you have coverage for the items on the list that follows. It can't hurt to ask, right? And it might really help financially.

NUTRITION

Many insurance companies will cover prenatal visits with a nutritionist, especially in twin pregnancies. If you are having trouble gaining enough weight, if you're gaining too quickly, or if you have been diagnosed with gestational diabetes, it's a good idea to make an appointment with a nutritionist.

NURSES

If you have a C-section, some insurance companies will cover a certain number of visiting nurse services to come to your house after the babies are born and check your incision.

BREAST-FEEDING SUPPLIES

Some insurance plans cover a visit with a lactation consultant, and some will also cover the cost of a breast pump (although it may not be the pump you like best). If they'll cover a pump, make sure to buy one even if you're planning on renting a hospital-grade pump or have no intention of nursing. Why not? You never know what will happen and you might end up using it.

Also, let's hope this doesn't happen, but depending on their conditions, if your children spend even one hour in the NICU, breast milk is then considered a medical necessity. In this case, your insurance company will most definitely cover your pump. Many NICUs have a standard letter at their desk that you need to submit to your insurance company along with your pump receipt. Check with your hospital for this paperwork. It will contain all of the codes you need to file the claim.

Thinking Ahead

In the very early stages of your pregnancy, your mind can spin with worry about all that lies ahead. Here are some practical tips for arming yourself with the right knowledge that will help ease your mind.

Easy Dos

There are a few more simple things that you can do now to prepare for your twins and check off your list. Your goal should be to have the majority of these items completed (or at least under way) by the time you pass twenty weeks of your pregnancy:

Tour the Hospital

Hospital tours sound pointless and boring, but when your babies are born, you are going to want to know where they are. You should know where the NICU and the nursery are, especially in relation to where you'll be in recovery. It's comforting to know where your children will be while you're recovering, and this will make it easier for your partner to go back and forth between you and the babies if need be. If your hospital doesn't offer a tour, which is unfortunately common these days, just go in and sneak around (but don't say that I told you to do that). If you feel uncomfortable sneaking around, call the hospital's public relations manager and see if something can be done.

Take a First Aid/Baby CPR Class

I cannot stress enough the importance of taking an infant CPR class. This needs to be done *while* you are expecting. If you wait till after the twinnies are here, you may not have the time. My daughter stopped breathing twice in our house, and we had to perform CPR on her, so I strongly recommend that every twin parent take an infant CPR course. Even if you never need it for your own children (and I hope this is the case), it's just good to know for somebody sitting next to you at a restaurant or another kid at the playground.

Also, make sure you go every year for your refresher course. Use the twins' birthday or your wedding anniversary as a reminder. Not only must you do this, but you should sign up anyone and everyone who is going to be spending time alone with the children, whether that's your mother, mother-in-law, nanny, or whoever. I don't care if your new caregiver says that she took a course last week; she can take a refresher class. It generally costs anywhere from thirty dollars to seventy-five dollars a class, depending on where you live, so just sign everyone up and you'll be able to sleep at night (for now).

Anticipate Bed Rest

Unless there is a specific medical concern, your doctor probably won't command you to go on bed rest, but please realize that once you hit thirty weeks, you may not want to do much. You may feel like throwing in the towel, kicking your feet up, and watching TV or reading a book. This is completely normal. At thirty-two weeks, your uterus will be the same size as a singleton mother's at forty weeks, so you will be understandably fatigued.

Expect to start making adjustments to your schedule at around the thirty-week mark. If you can stop working, go for it. If you have to keep working, find a way to take a nap in your office or keep your feet up under your desk. If your job requires you to be on your feet, you just might want to stop even sooner, depending on how you feel. If you do end up on bed rest, check your short-term disability benefits. If you can collect disability payments, do it. Every penny counts.

Bottom line: Enjoy as much rest as you can before those babies arrive.

Know the Signs of Preterm Labor

The signs of preterm labor vary from pregnancy to pregnancy. What might have been a harmless symptom for your sister may not be for you. Speak with your doctor about what you should look out for in regard to preterm labor. If you Google "signs of preterm labor," you'll find hundreds of symptoms, from stomach cramping to heavy spotting. These are all true, but I tell my Twiniversity students to call your doctor if you have:

- Any excessive cramping
- Any spotting (of any color)
- Any unusual discharge
- Any lower back pain
- Any unexplained diarrhea
- Any contractions (Any! Even if they aren't steady or strong, call the doc.)
- Any pelvic pressure

But the No. 1 thing I tell my students is to trust your instincts. Don't feel funny calling the doctor. You won't regret it, so if you are feeling "off" or just not like yourself, call your doctor, describe your symptoms, and let them make the call on if you should come in or not. Also, one thing you should definitely do to help prevent preterm labor is to go to the dentist. Gingivitis can be a trigger. Have a regular checkup and a cleaning early in your pregnancy. I'll talk more about preterm labor in chapter 2.

What Not to Do

What you don't do while preparing for your twins' arrival is just as important as what you do do. Here are just a few activities that you should just discontinue or never start, to save time and frustration.

Don't Google "Micro Preemies"

Don't be tempted to start doing research on preemies and preemie issues and all of that jazz. If you ever need that information, you will be able to get it then. You don't need to scare yourself silly in the meantime.

Don't Take a Lamaze Class

This may sound counterintuitive, but remember that what makes sense for singleton parents doesn't always make sense for us. You are almost definitely not going to have the beautiful, candlelit natural birth that they teach you about in Lamaze classes, and paying to hear about it might make you get a little upset. If you want the experience and education, a great option is to check out the DVD *Laugh and Learn about Childbirth* by Sheri Bayles. You can watch this six-parter in the comfort of your own living room. However, if you want to round out your pregnancy experience and always dreamed of taking this type of course, go right ahead and enjoy it. Perhaps your hospital has a specific birthing class just for parents of multiples or you can ask the Lamaze instructor for a private class. There are options, but if your time and budget are limited, don't feel bad skipping this class entirely.

Sometimes I feel like a unicorn in the twin world when folks find out that I had a vaginal delivery. Here in New York City it's fairly uncommon, and scheduled C-sections seem to be the growing trend for twin moms around the globe. Considering that I did have a vaginal delivery, I want to assure you that no matter how many classes you take or skip, your body will do its job come "showtime." I'm still in awe of how my entire being just went into autopilot to help push the babies out. It's almost as if there is an inner cavewoman waiting to come out, and the birth of your children is the time that she truly shines. Rest assured that millions of women are having children around the globe today. Some of them have taken Lamaze and some haven't, but they will have a beautiful end result regardless. If you end up skipping a birthing class, your birthing team will be right there to coach you through every breath. Good luck!

Don't Neglect Your Spouse

Sure, it's all about you and the two babies that you're growing (and of course that's how it should be), but don't forget about the person who got you into this mess in the first place. Your partner is busy adjusting to the idea of being a parent of twins, too, so make sure to set aside time to talk about how you're both feeling. Also continue going on date nights until you're too tired to go anywhere but the couch, and then just have date nights right there.

Don't Push Yourself

Honestly, growing two infants from scratch is more than most people accomplish in a lifetime, and you're doing it at once! Give yourself a break. Take any help that is offered to you, whether it's from your husband to do the dishes or a coworker to grab you a sandwich at lunchtime. You need to rest and your babies need you to rest. Lower your expectations of what you can do and start to slow down now.

> **From the MOM Squad:** *"We were ecstatic. We struggled for ten years to have children and were so hopeful for one child. When we found out we were having two, we felt so blessed. I turned to my husband and said, 'We need another crib.'"* —Jill L.

Don't Listen to Horror Stories

I wish there were a way for me to prevent anyone from saying anything ever again along the lines of, "Wow, twins!" "That will be so hard for you."

"How will you manage?" "My friend Sheila had twins and she didn't sleep more than an hour a night for the first two years!" I'll go ahead and assume that these people mean well, but that doesn't really make this stuff any easier for you to hear. Completely ignore these comments as much as you can. You will manage just like all of the twin mamas who came before you, and you will be fine. Cut people like this off with a quick, "I'm sure I'll manage fine, thanks."

Celebrations Times Two

You can't finish mentally preparing for twins without a little celebration! Twin baby showers can be twice as much fun as singleton showers. If you have a great friend or family member who wants to organize a party, definitely take them up on it. You're going to need a lot of gear when the babies arrive, and showers are a great way to start gathering together what you need. See chapter 5 for a full list of must-have gear. If your culture allows it, I strongly recommend that you schedule your babies' shower somewhere between your twenty-sixth and thirtieth week of pregnancy. You don't want to have it too soon, but you do want to have it soon enough that you'll be able to enjoy it without being too exhausted during the festivities.

If you do end up having a shower, here's a tip that will save you a huge amount of time: let each of your guests address their own thank-you card! Give everyone a note card envelope and ask them to write their name and address on it. For me, this was a real time saver. Since my twinnies came early, I was very late with my thank-you cards. Everyone told me it wasn't necessary, but it was important for me to make sure that my friends and family knew how thankful I really was. So instead of traditional, individualized thank-you notes, I wrote this poem and sent it to each guest:

Surprise, we came early!
So our parents' "thank-you"s are late
We hope you understand
That now they have a lot on their plate

They need to feed us and change us
At least a dozen times a day
And with two that takes a lot of time
We're a lot of work they say

It's actually two in the morning
As our mommy writes this poem
'Cause that's the only time there's peace
In our humble little home

So thank you very much,
For the gifts, good wishes, and prayers
We feel so blessed to have such great support
From our family and friends who truly care.

Pregnancy Checklist

Here is a handy list of everything that you need to get done over the next nine months, broken down by trimester. Don't panic; just take a breath and get started checking things off.

First Trimester
— Start a video, online, or paper journal
— Join Twiniversity and another twins group in your area
— Research hospitals
— Stop smoking and drinking
— Attend a local twins club meeting
— Do Kegel exercises
— Plan babies' budget
— Take some photos of your growing belly
— Find out your company's maternity leave and your partner's paternity leave policies
— Consult with your doctor about any medications you're taking

__Find the right obstetrician

__Start a savings plan (more on this in chapter 4)

__Look for a new home (if necessary)

__Start a pregnancy workout

Second Trimester

__Remove wedding rings and other jewelry in case of swelling

__Move into new home (if necessary)

__Paint the nursery

__Attend a local twins club meeting

__Take your hospital tour

__Pack your hospital bag (see pages 125–126)

__Plan homecoming outfits for the twins

__Do Kegel exercises

__Call your insurance company to check coverage

__Schedule prenatal massage

__Go on a baby moon (a minivacation with your spouse before the babies arrive)

__Don't forget to take photos of your growing belly

__Learn the signs of preterm labor

__Decide if you'll circumcise if you're expecting boys

__Create a phone and e-mail list to alert people after the babies have arrived

__Research cord blood donation or storage

__Find a lactation consultant in your area

__Register for your gear

__Prepare your pets

__Buy a new car if necessary

__Plan your baby shower

__Send your baby shower invitations

__Set up automatic bill pay for your utilities and credit cards

__Update your will

__Pick out your birth announcements

__Hire household help to clean if you are not up to it

__Find a baby nurse

__Interview prenatal doulas if you'd like to have one

__Attend a Lamaze class or watch a DVD

__Create a first aid kit if you don't have one

__Go to the dentist

__Share the good news with your family

__Share the good news with your coworkers and boss

__Check your company's disability policy

__Have a baby shower

Third Trimester

__Install car seats and get them inspected

__Attend a local twins club meeting

__Do your Kegel exercises

__Don't forget to take photos of your growing belly

__Wash and put away the babies' clothing

__Attend a breast-feeding class

__Cook and freeze nutritious meals for after the babies have arrived

__Figure out who's going to be part of your labor team

__Assemble cribs

__Get your nursery in order

__Decorate your nursery

__Pick out names

__Interview pediatricians

__Send your baby shower thank-you cards

__Childproof your home

__Buy life insurance

__Find a nanny

__Prepare your birth plan

__Shop for nursing bras

__Figure out your new work schedule

__Discuss with your obstetrician the circumstances under which he or she is willing to perform a vaginal delivery vs. a C-section

__Buy diapers and wipes

__Prepare for the possibility of bed rest

CHAPTER 2

the double pregnancy

. . . .

I F YOU OR SOMEONE YOU LOVE IS PREGNANT WITH TWINS (AND WHY else would you be reading this book?), you've probably already noticed many of the differences between a twin pregnancy and a singleton pregnancy. While the biological process is more or less the same, having two little beings in a womb that was really built for one complicates things more than a little bit. This chapter is not meant to scare you. The vast majority of twin pregnancies go off without a hitch, producing two beautiful and perfectly healthy babies. But complications and uncomfortable annoyances do come up in all pregnancies, and there are some specific issues that only present themselves in twin pregnancies (lucky us!), so it is important to be informed.

The most common concern in a twin pregnancy is preterm labor, which results in the babies being born too soon. It is simply more difficult for mothers of twins to carry their babies to term. While this is a valid concern, be reassured that with modern medical practices, even micro preemies who would not have been considered viable just a decade or two ago can now thrive and go on to live completely normal lives. My babies were born at thirty-four weeks and spent weeks in the NICU, and I am very relieved to tell you that today they are healthy, thriving seven-year-olds. Your twins are much more than likely to be fine, even if they do come early.

This chapter will address all of the ways that a twin pregnancy differs from a singleton pregnancy, the discomforts that particularly plague us, and my best advice for managing each of these issues for the maximum health and comfort of you and your babies. Put those feet up and keep reading!

Double Duty at the Doctor

You may have already noticed that we twin mamas see our doctors a lot more than the average singleton mother. Because of the inherent increased risks in a twin pregnancy, you will see your physician an average of thirty percent more than a singleton mom does. Yes, it is a pain to drag your pregnant self back and forth to the office so many times, but try to see this as a good thing. First of all, it's always reassuring to hear those two heartbeats or to see those two little beings in an ultrasound. And it helps you start to bond with them very early on.

However, as you may already know, a simple doctor's visit can be a positive experience or a major headache, depending on many factors that have nothing to do with the babies themselves! Here are my top tips for getting the most out of your appointments so that you can relax and focus on gawking at the image of the two little miracles you created on the screen.

Start a Medical Journal

It's a good idea to buy a new journal to use during your pregnancy as a resource. When questions come up between doctor visits, you may be 100 percent sure that you'll remember to ask when the time comes, but I promise that you will forget to ask at least one thing. Have a specific place to

TWINIVERSITY TIP: MAKE FRIENDS IN HIGH PLACES

The person in charge of your doctor's schedule is actually much more important than your actual physician (in some ways). Your doctor will see whoever is in the room, but the scheduler is the one who gets you in there. Get to know the person at the front desk. Learn their kids' names, bring them a cup of coffee or a pastry, or splurge on a small gift card. Wink, wink. These little things can go a really, really long way.

write questions down and run through them with your doctor and then write down the answers (because you might forget those, too).

Call Yourself

If you're not into pen and paper, you can use your phone to make a voice memo for yourself or even call your own voice mail and just leave it running for the entire visit with your OB. This is actually great for partners who can't make it to the appointment, because they can listen to the whole visit later and feel like they were there.

Get E-mail Access

Even though we e-mail about everything else in life, many of us are so accustomed to calling the doctor with every question we have that we never consider using e-mail for this purpose. But I encourage you to get your doctor's address. E-mail is the perfect medium for random questions and concerns that aren't urgent but can't really wait until your next visit. If you're up in the middle of the night worrying that you may have caught a random virus the last time you took the bus, just e-mail your doctor and get it off your chest. Once it's out there, you can stop worrying about it. If your doctor doesn't have an e-mail address (or doesn't feel comfortable giving it to patients), there's probably someone in the office who does, whether it's a colleague or a nurse who can answer routine questions.

Alternatively, if your doctor texts, then text when you have questions. A lot of physicians have their cell phones on hand all the time and will answer you right away via text, while they might wait until the end of the day to check their office voice mail.

Ask the Dumb Questions

If the doctor says something that you don't understand, don't just nod as if you completely get it just because you're embarrassed to admit that you don't. This is not your nineteenth pregnancy, so how should you know? Go ahead and ask. No one is judging you. Don't forget that nurses are an excellent resource for information, too, and they might have more time to spend with you than your doctor.

Get Copies of All Your Test Results

Any time your doctor's office calls with the results of a test, ask them to fax or e-mail you a copy of the results. This is great for your general records, insurance claims, and a million other reasons. Just start a "test results" folder and file everything in there. Even better, take a picture of the test results with your phone so that you have them with you at all times. This will be a lifesaver if you ever have to visit the hospital for any reason. You can show them these pictures of your results instead of waiting for them to get copies from your doctor.

Record Your Sonogram

This may sound crazy, but when you go to the doctor's office for your next visit, ask if you can record your sonogram. You can bring a blank DVD, a thumb drive, or a VHS tape (depending on the doctor's equipment). Truthfully, the only reason that we still have a VHS player in my house is that my sonogram is on a VHS tape and my kids love to watch it. They get a huge kick out of seeing themselves really living in there, and of course I love to watch it, too. This is just a fun idea, but it can be really great to have down the road and it's something you can't do over after they are born.

Pregnancy Discomforts: Yes, You Will Be Tired!

Twin mamas suffer from many of the same problems as moms of singletons, ranging from simple discomforts to life-threatening emergencies. We are just so lucky that the discomforts start earlier and are often more severe. Count yourself doubly blessed for these all too common pregnancy complaints.

Fatigue

The No. 1 complaint of all twin mamas is fatigue. If you're someone who used to burn the midnight oil and now you're passing out on the couch at 9 o'clock, just throw in the towel, man. Don't feel bad about it. I always laugh when I hear women who are carrying twins ask, "Why am I so tired?" You're building not one, but two humans in there. That's why. Go to bed already. Go to bed now. You have my full permission.

Hemorrhoids

Well, this sure is a fun one, isn't it? It's the best! Look, a lot of us get these during a twin pregnancy. Don't feel weird about it. It's fine. You get them because your body needs so many nutrients to build those two humans inside of you that it squeezes every little last bit of useful goodness from the foods you eat. So you have very little coming out the other end, am I right? This is one of the most common pregnancy side effects and it happens even more with twins.

The best solution to this one is to eat. You can take fiber supplements until the cows come home, but that's not going to help as much as just eating whole, unprocessed food. Don't be shy about it. If you need to eat a whole bag of baby carrots, do it. Nobody's going to look at you funny. If you need to consume an entire pot of lentil soup, you just go ahead and eat it. Eat real, whole foods and drink water like it's your job, like it's a reality show challenge for you to drink as much water as you can. Shoot for a minimum of a gallon of water a day. That's right—a gallon. Don't complain about it. It's not gasoline; it's water. It's good for the hemorrhoid issue and it's good for the babies. (I'll talk more about that later.)

Insomnia

Are you wondering why you can't sleep anymore? Mother Nature is just getting you ready for life with newborn twins. If you're up from 3 a.m. to 5 a.m., just know that that's probably going to be feeding time. At least you'll be prepared. Embrace your new life as an insomniac. Get up, read a book, play on the computer, and wait until you're ready to go back to sleep. Don't just lie there and toss and turn, or you'll really aggravate your partner for no reason. If you are tossing and turning a lot, you might just not be comfortable in bed anymore. I'm not saying partners shouldn't share in the full pregnancy experience, I'm just saying they need sleep, too. If you have to move out to the living room, it's okay. Try to sleep on a recliner or on the couch, or perhaps try to take the couch cushions into bed with you. It may be worth the investment to purchase a full body pillow. You can cradle it under your bump and tuck it between your arms and legs, as well. It's worth a try if too much sleep is getting away from you.

Reflux

Isn't pregnancy a joy? If you are suffering from reflux during your pregnancy, just Tums the day away, with your doctor's permission, of course. When I was pregnant, I ate orange Tums like they were M&M's. Just shove them down and don't think about it. Another option is to try eating almonds before going to bed. Almonds neutralize stomach acids, so they just might work. Try sleeping in a more upright position, too. In our family, my little old Italian grandmother Anna told me to take a teaspoon of apple cider vinegar when heartburn hits. Truth be told, this has worked 100 percent of the time for me and many of my other Twiniversity families.

Swelling

This is another good one. You might get really swollen, probably starting in the second trimester. There will be a lot more volume in your body—a lot more blood and water—so don't be alarmed if you start to resemble the Stay Puft Marshmallow Man. However, there is such a thing as bad swelling. You can tell the difference this way: if you press your fingertips into the swollen part of your body and it remains indented where your fingers were, tell your doctor. Otherwise, just lie in bed with your feet up. There's really not much else you can do. But it's always a good idea to call your physician's office if you notice swelling and let them decide if they want to have you come in to assess your swelling. Severe cases could be a sign of preeclampsia (see page 36).

If you have a toe ring or an ankle bracelet, you should really take those puppies off now. You don't want to wake up one morning and wonder what happened to your toe ring. Also, I hate to say it, but it's not a bad idea to take your wedding and engagement rings off as well. I know it kind of sucks, but look on the bright side—you can start dating again; no one will know you're married! Seriously, though, take them off and put them someplace safe. In fact, I would write down where you put them. Send yourself and your spouse an e-mail with the location! It would really stink to forget where your rings were when you can finally wear them again.

Back Pain

Singleton moms get a lot of back pain, too, but ours is worse (yay!). Your abs will stretch to their maximum capacity, you lose a lot of strength there, and your back has to compensate. A number of moms have found relief for back pain in acupuncture or chiropractic treatments. If you want to try this, make sure that you go to someone who has all of the proper licenses. It's a good idea to get referrals from other moms. Another good idea is to invest in a pregnancy belt. True, they aren't the sexiest undergarments in the world, but you'll be comfortable. It's worth a try if you are really suffering.

Incontinence

This is such a fun list, isn't it? I have to tell you, the absolute best thing about being a mom is sneezing and peeing on myself. Seriously, this experience is right up there with the first time I held my twins. (Yes, I'm kidding.) This happens because we have a lot of weight on our bladders. The only solution here is to Kegel forever. A Kegel exercise is used to strengthen the pelvic floor and helps wonderfully during pregnancy (so you don't sneeze and pee on yourself), assists with muscles used in a vaginal birth, and helps your lady parts bounce back after delivery. If you have never done Kegels before, the next time you are in the ladies' room, stop the flow of urine midway. Let your urine flow again and then stop it again. Your Kegel muscle is what you used to make that happen. Keep starting and stopping your flow of urine until you are able to isolate that muscle so you can flex it again later. After you are out of the ladies' room, try to isolate that muscle again. Can you do it? If not, wait until you have to go to the restroom again and try once more. Once you are successful in flexing your Kegel muscle, start your "reps." Try to hold your pelvic floor muscle for ten seconds straight. You may not be able to hold it for even three seconds at first; you'll have to work up to it. Once you get there, try to do three sets of 10 reps (for ten seconds each) a few times a day. These few minutes out of your day will save you a lot of trouble in the long run. It's not always guaranteed to work, but it's definitely worth a shot. Do some Kegels every time you think of it. Do some now; I won't tell anyone. It's worth a little effort so that you are not sneezing and peeing on yourself later on in life.

Round Ligament Pain

To put it simply, the ligament that holds your uterus in place is going to stretch quite a bit, and it's going to hurt. You may get stuck in the middle of a store and not be able to take another step. This is motherhood. This is what we signed up for. Any time anything like this happened to me, my sister would remind me that I paid extra for this thanks to my IVF treatment. And it was all worth every penny.

> **From the MOM Squad:** *"I was least prepared for how much I actually enjoyed pregnancy. After hearing about and reading about all the discomforts of pregnancy and all the things that can go wrong with a twin pregnancy, I think I became overly focused on the downside. Yes, it was difficult and uncomfortable and scary, but it was also amazing and wonderful. I gained a whole new appreciation for my body because of what it was able to do during pregnancy."* —Cynthia M.

Morning Sickness

If you are already suffering from the nausea and vomiting that comes with morning sickness, you are not alone. Half of all pregnant women suffer from morning sickness, and twin mamas experience it even more, due to elevated levels of human chronic gonadotropin. This is the same hormone that confirms your pregnancy in the beginning. Rising estrogen and progesterone levels contribute to morning sickness, too, and being pregnant with twins causes higher than normal levels of those hormones. Lucky us! Rest assured that in most cases symptoms subside as these hormones level out early in your second trimester. Until then, here are some tips for dealing with one of the most unpleasant parts of a twin pregnancy.

Avoid Scent Triggers

During pregnancy, your increased sensitivity to smells can bring on nausea and vomiting. Avoid cooking with spices that trigger these feelings and avoid busy restaurants with poor ventilation.

Avoid Food Triggers

Try not to eat greasy, high-fat, high-sugar, and acidic foods that can irritate your stomach. Focus on eating bland foods until your morning sickness passes.

Drink Water

It's extra important to stay hydrated during a twin pregnancy, especially if you're throwing up and losing fluids that way. Some moms say that adding lemon or mint to their water helped them keep it down.

Try Ginger

Ginger is widely known to help settle the stomach—that's why you're supposed to drink ginger ale when you are sick. But ginger comes in many forms—candied ginger, ginger chews, capsules, tea, or good old ginger ale. Try any and all of these to help alleviate your morning sickness.

Eat

Though the last thing you want to do right now is eat, it's important that you try. Sometimes, getting too hungry in the first place makes you feel even more nauseous. Eat smaller meals throughout the day to keep your tummy full and to prevent acids from building up. Eating something before getting out of bed in the morning sometimes helps. Try keeping some crackers in your nightstand. Some moms have said that sucking on hard candies such as cinnamon candies, sour lemon candies, and Lifesavers had helped alleviate their morning sickness. It's definitely worth a try, right?

Use Supplements

Vitamin B_6 and B_{12} supplements have also been known to help with nausea and vomiting. Talk to your doctor before trying these to make sure it's safe and get a recommended dosage.

Take It Slow

Sudden changes like getting out of bed or standing up too fast may bring on a wave of nausea. Change positions gradually.

Get Meds

There are prescription drugs that you can take if your morning sickness persists despite these efforts. Talk to your doctor if you can't keep anything down and you are worried about becoming dehydrated.

More Severe Issues

Yes, some conditions popping up during a twin pregnancy are cause for a little more concern. Rest assured that, while these conditions may be more serious, they will not harm you or your babies in the vast majority of cases if treated properly. Just educate yourself so that you can recognize the symptoms early and talk to your doctor if you have any concerns.

Gestational Diabetes

Gestational diabetes is more common in mothers of twins than in singleton mothers. Women who are diagnosed with gestational diabetes are at a higher risk of developing type 2 diabetes later in life. That said, the biggest risk associated with gestational diabetes is delivering a large baby and needing a C-section, which isn't much of a risk for twin moms because most twins are not big babies. If you're diagnosed with gestational diabetes, don't panic but do realize that you're going to have to make some adjustments. This is temporary and crucial for your kids' health—both short and long term—so try to summon your inner "healthy eater" for the next few months! Also keep in mind that this is not your fault or something you've brought on.

Your doctor may send you to a nutritionist or dietitian to review the dietary recommendations that will help you keep your blood sugar in the normal range. Yes, that probably means no more cookies and ice cream, but you should not be starving yourself! You will need to try to find a way to eat on a regular schedule and check your blood sugar often. If your doctor gives you the okay to exercise, do it! This will also help to even out your blood sugar.

Preeclampsia

This, too, is more common during twin pregnancies. Experts still don't know exactly what causes this condition to occur, but it is marked by high blood pressure, protein in the urine, and severe swelling. Untreated, it can lead to early delivery and even become fatal, so this is something to take seriously. If you see any sudden swelling, call your doctor right away.

Placental Abruption

This is when the placenta detaches from the uterine wall prior to delivery. It is a very rare but serious condition that is also more common in twin pregnancies (though still rare). If you experience a partial abruption (when the placenta only detaches partially from the uterus), you will likely be put on bed rest, and depending on how far along your pregnancy is, you may have a C-section to remove the twins before they are put at risk. In the case of a total separation, delivery (often via C-section) is the safest course of action. The most common sign of placental abruption is vaginal bleeding, so call your doctor if you experience this.

Placenta Previa

This is when the placenta forms on the lower portion of the uterus and partially or fully covers the cervix. Twins mamas are, you guessed it, at a higher risk for placenta previa. If you are diagnosed with this, you should know that it often corrects itself as the pregnancy progresses. In other cases, the mother is put on bed rest to try and avoid preterm labor. In the vast majority of cases, the babies are delivered without any problems, often via C-section to avoid the risk of bleeding.

Identical Twin-Specific Issues

Lucky mothers of identical twins not only have to deal with all of the traditional pregnancy concerns, but also the additional twin issues and a few complications made especially for them! Because the babies share a

> ◎/◎
>
> ### Types of Twins Cheat Sheet
>
> - Monozygotic: Twins formed from a single fertilized egg that split. This split egg forms two embryos and creates identical twins.
> - Dizygotic: Twins formed from two separate fertilized eggs that grew into embryos. These are known as fraternal twins.

placenta in identical twin pregnancies, there can be complications that arise. Please keep in mind that they are rare, even in monozygotic (twin) pregnancies.

Selective Intrauterine Growth Restriction (SIUGR)

SIUGR affects 10 percent of pregnancies with monochorionic (shared placenta) multiples. This issue arises when the nourishment of your placenta is not shared equally between the twins.

In other words, your twins are already bad at sharing and aren't receiving equal nutrition from the placenta. This may result in poor nourishment for one of the twins, causing overall poor fetal growth.

Twin to Twin Transfusion Syndrome (TTTS)

TTTS is a disease of the placenta. This occurs when blood moves from one twin to the other via the umbilical cord. The twin who loses blood (the donor twin) and the one who receives it (the recipient twin) are both negatively affected, the extent of which depends on the severity of the transfusion. This occurs in one in seven monochorionic twin pregnancies. Left untreated, the mortality rate is near 100 percent.

Rest assured that we have had many Twiniversity families who have very successfully delivered healthy monochorionic twins. Not every pregnancy will result in issues. These topics are not here to scare you, just to educate you.

> **Note from Dad:** *"At first my wife was very nervous about having twins and I would try to reassure her that we would be alright financially, emotionally, and physically. I would attend as many doctor's appointments with her as I could to be there for her and we would get information together. I just tried to listen and participate in every step of the process."* —Eric B.

If you are diagnosed with one of these syndromes or any fetal-related syndrome, reach out to Fetal Health Foundation. They are an organization that was created and run by several families around the country who have dealt with TTTS, with varying outcomes. The foundation serves as a liaison between families diagnosed with intrauterine fetal syndromes like TTTS, amniotic band syndrome (ABS), hypoplastic left heart syndrome (HLHS), lower urinary tract obstruction (LUTO), and many others. They offer support through family matching, online forums, bereavement counseling, and travel grants when travel for lifesaving treatment is immediate and necessary. Fetal Health Foundation serves to empower parents with knowledge and information in advocating for their unborn twins. You can learn more at www.fetalhealthfoundation.org.

Eating for Three

First of all, this is not the time to diet. Honestly, it might be hard for you to make the mental shift from being calorie-conscious to consciously eating more calories. It will hopefully help for you to know that studies have shown that the more weight a twin mama gains during her first two trimesters, the more likely she is to carry her twins to term. Gaining the right amount of weight throughout your pregnancy is something that you can actually control, unlike so many elements of your pregnancy, so this is something that you can focus on doing right. It isn't something to take lightly; the health of your children depends on what you eat, when you eat, and how much you eat. Here are all of the details you need to know about eating for three.

Weight Gain

I asked ob-gyn and twin mom Dr. Barbara Deli for her expert recommendations about how much weight a twin mama should gain throughout her pregnancy. Here's what she had to say:

"The reality is that the right amount of weight to gain is different for everyone and everyone gains weight at a different pace. The Institute of Medicine has come up with weight gain recommendations based on your starting weight. Use these only as general guidelines.

* Normal-weight women—37 to 54 pounds
* Overweight women—31 to 50 pounds
* Obese women—25 to 42 pounds

"If you're eating comfortably and at times don't gain much weight, don't stress about it. Remember that the babies are very efficient at taking all the nutrition they need from you. Many women struggle to eat well and gain very little (or lose weight) in the first trimester. This is temporary and your body will make up for it later when the nausea subsides. If you go week after week without gaining weight, talk to your doctor or a nutritionist about your day-to-day diet.

"Gaining more than you (or your doctor) expect can slightly increase your chance of pregnancy complications like diabetes and high blood pressure. Studies of twin pregnancies have shown that upper limits of weight gain in pregnancy are less important to worry about in twins than in singleton pregnancies. The more weight women gain in pregnancy, even above the recommendations, the bigger the babies are at birth. Higher birth weights are a good thing in most twins, especially premature ones!"

Calories Count

In general, your daily calorie consumption should be approximately 2,300 to 2,700 calories. That is a lot. Come on, kids, it's awesome. This is your chance to live it up, so dream big. Eat several times a day. Eat three meals and at least three snacks a day. You should be eating something at least every couple of hours. Grab a snack right now! This is literally your job now.

Protein Power

Nearly as important as getting enough calories is eating enough protein. Protein is like the little building blocks that will create your babies, and your body needs a lot of it. You need at least 130 grams of protein a day. That is a lot of chicken salad sandwiches and peanut butter. Make protein a priority. The best way to do this is to look at your plate and eat the protein first, and then finish anything else you can stomach. If proteins aren't sitting well, try black beans, or high-protein grains like quinoa. If you are a vegetarian, check with your doctor or think about seeing a nutritionist to make sure that you are meeting your protein needs throughout your pregnancy.

Daily Vitamins

It is important to make sure that you are taking your prenatal daily vitamins. If you are tired of paying for your daily vitamins, when you go to the doctor's office, ask them to give you a boatload of samples. They will give them to you. I don't want you to be shy about anything like that ever again. Every time you go to the doctor's office, just ask for whatever you want. The birth of your twins can cost almost a hundred grand between your hospital stay, the babies' hospital stays, plus every freaking specialist in the universe who is going to come witness your birth and probably bill for it. I think you deserve some free vitamins.

Water

I mentioned this before, but it's worth bringing up again. You need to drink at least a gallon of water a day not only to prevent hemorrhoids and all that fun stuff, but also to ward off dehydration and preterm labor. If your body gets too dehydrated, your muscles can tighten and cramp, and this can be confused with labor pains, so it is crucial that you remain properly hydrated throughout your twin pregnancy. You should never be without a bottle of water. It's worth it to invest in a good refillable bottle. Know how many times you have to refill it to meet your daily water quota. Try better than your best to drink every drop. It's important.

What Not to Eat

There are some foods (and drinks) that all mommies-to-be should avoid. Here is a quick list of the foods that doctors most commonly suggest pregnant women stay away from. Discuss these with your health care professional, as opinions on these things are constantly changing!

Raw Fish, Eggs, and Meat

The raw foods themselves aren't dangerous, but they run the risk of containing bacteria that can harm your twins. I know that pregnant Japanese women eat sushi nonstop, but most doctors in this country suggest that you avoid it. If there is something you are craving but you are not sure if there might be a health risk, ask your health care professional. As always, it's best to err on the side of caution.

High-Mercury Seafood

Your twins eat what you eat, and so high levels of mercury can damage their developing brains and bodies. High-mercury seafoods include shark, swordfish, and tilefish. Tuna has moderate amounts of mercury and should be eaten only once a week. (This goes for nursing moms, too!)

Unpasteurized Milk and Cheese

Unpasteurized milk and soft cheeses such as Brie, feta, and Gorgonzola may contain bacteria listeria, which has been linked to miscarriage risk. Read your packages carefully!

Caffeine

This one is controversial for obvious reasons! Many twin mamas can't handle coffee during pregnancy, anyway, because of morning sickness and heartburn. Plus, high levels of caffeine have been linked to miscarriage, premature birth, and low birth weights, which are of utmost concern for twins. If you can't live without your morning cup of joe, you should be able to safely drink one cup a day, but you should discuss it with your doctor.

Alcohol

No known amount of alcohol is considered safe during pregnancy, so it is best to avoid it altogether. Drinking alcohol during pregnancy can lead to fetal alcohol syndrome and other developmental delays. If you drank before you knew you were pregnant, start abstaining the moment the pregnancy is confirmed!

Signs of Preterm Labor

I'm not a medical doctor, I've never played one on TV, and I don't want to be one. (It's way too much school for me.) But I have been through this and heard from enough twin mamas to know the signs backward and forward. Call your ob-gyn if you feel like you're getting your period, have any kind of cramping in your uterus, or have any kind of discharge. I don't care if it's yellow, red, pink, purple, or blue—call your doctor. Remember that if you haven't had a child before, you don't really know what labor feels like. (Lucky you!)

I'll tell you the truth—labor pains are so bad that you will know for sure what they are. If you feel like you need to bite on to a belt with all your might or that your midsection is being compressed by some medieval torture device, then you're in labor. So if you feel any kind of intense pain, call your doctor right away. But early labor isn't nearly as intense, so if you feel any cramping whatsoever that is consistent you should go ahead and call your doctor, too.

The truth is, your instincts are going to steer you in the right direction when it comes to understanding something is wrong. I really mean this from the bottom of my heart. Even if you feel nothing but the hairs of the back of your neck sticking up and you don't feel right, call your doctor. Always err on the side of caution. Don't stress about it, just go in and get checked as much as you need to. Become best friends with the nurses at the hospital. The more they see you, the better treatment you're going to get anyway.

My story proves it. My husband and I were getting ready to go to a party on a boat. I had bought a new dress. I had to wear slippers because none of my shoes fit anymore, but whatever—I was going to rock that new dress with the slippers. But right before we were going to leave, I started to feel like something wasn't right. I called my doctor and it turned out that I was in labor. It was real, legit labor, but I didn't feel anything. It was just my gut telling me that something was up, and I was right. The medical team was able to treat and stabilize my contractions. I was eventually discharged and told to take it easy. I did just that. I was able to make it a few more blissful weeks with the babies tucked safely inside my growing belly.

Don't worry if your doctor hates you if you "cry wolf" too many times. The health of you and your babies is paramount. If you have a question or you're worried, call and just run it by them. Really trust those instincts. Women have been having children for a few years now, and your body will never steer you in the wrong direction. Now, if you're feeling pain, but it's a little irregular, it might be just gas or something. Go to bed, lie down on your left side, drink a glass of water, and see what happens. If it goes away, then you're fine, but if not, go ahead and call your doctor, even if it's 2 o'clock in the morning.

Bed Rest

Many twin mamas live in fear of bed rest for their entire pregnancies, but some never have to spend one day with our feet up. (Well, under doctor's orders, that is.) Others panic when their physician finally says that it's time to go on bed rest. First of all, being put on bed rest does not necessarily mean that your twins' health is in immediate danger, so there's no need to panic. Find out why your doctor wants you to go on bed rest. Have you started having contractions? Is your blood pressure too high? Has your cervix started to dilate? Is your job just too taxing for your body? Is your amniotic fluid leaking? Knowing why you've been asked to go on bed rest should alleviate some of your fears or at least put things in perspective. Most often, your doctor wants to make sure you are taking care of yourself and is putting you on bed rest in an effort to keep your babies safe in your uterus for as long as possible.

If you have been put on bed rest and it is for a legitimate reason, try your best to see this as a good thing. First of all, by resting you are giving your babies their best shot at a healthy start in life, so you can feel good about that. Plus, once those twins are born you are really going to wish you had more time to rest, so try to enjoy having doctor's orders to rest up! Here are some tips to make your time in bed as comfortable and enjoyable as possible.

TWINIVERSITY TIP

If you are carrying monoamniotic twins (identical twins that share one amniotic sac and share a placenta), you might be put on bed rest sooner than the rest of us because your pregnancy is inherently higher risk. It's easier said than done, but try not to worry too much! Your medical team will keep a close eye on you, and we've had many Twiniversity members successfully give birth to perfectly healthy monoamniotic twins.

Find Out Your Specific Restrictions

Can you sit up? Can you take a shower? Can you eat dinner at the table? Can you run small errands (to the drugstore, to get the kids from school, etc.)? How limited are you? Not all "bed rest" prescriptions are alike. I once held an online Twiniversity class with a mom who had to lie flat on her back with her camera above her. She'd been put on the most severe type of bed rest, but she rocked it out and has a beautiful set of triplets to prove it.

Get a Lap Desk

If your doctor allows you to sit up, it's great to have a hard surface to put pens and paper or your laptop, or anything you want nearby, on. Go old school and think about getting a "breakfast in bed" tray, which will give you more stability than a true lap desk. Plus, the sides will stabilize the tray when you have to adjust yourself a thousand times a day.

Turn on the Lights

Make sure there is a lamp close by so you can reach and adjust it yourself. If you are on strict bed rest, look into attaching a motion sensor to your light so that you can turn it on and off while lying down.

Break Out the Baby Monitor

If you hate yelling across the house, set up the baby monitor on your nightstand so that you can tell your husband to bring you another pint of Cherry Garcia before he comes back upstairs. Texting will also work. Video chat will also work wonders for feeling connected to the outside world.

Keep Snacks Close By

Get a minifridge for your bedroom and stock it with fresh fruit and veggies and plenty of water. Again, you need to eat like it's your job, and you shouldn't be getting up and down for snacks.

Keep Up Your Beauty Routine

Your skin and lips will get dry, so keep some lotion and lip balm handy. If you are feeling down in the dumps, add some lip gloss and mascara. Sometimes little touches like this can help you feel like yourself again.

Keep Your Remote Handy

Even if you've never been into TV, bed rest is the time to indulge. If there's nothing on the tube, experiment with different streaming options like Netflix, iTunes, Hulu, and even HBO Go. It's worth the money to keep your sanity. My pregnancy was filled with old *Arrested Development* and *Angel* episodes. Consider watching an entire sitcom or drama series that you didn't have time to commit to before. Time is on your side here, so go for it!

Keep a Journal

Spend some time on bed rest writing letters to your twins. Write down stories about your childhood and what you hope theirs will be like. Tell them about the day you met their dad and ask him to write down his side of the story. It will be fun for your twins to read later on in life. Get a head start on your baby books. Now's the best time!

Go Online

While you're surfing the Net, go ahead and Google your ex-boyfriend. Find out where your old college roommate lives and what became of your best friend from the third grade. Join Ancestry.com and learn about your family history so that you can share it with your twins. The addictive power of the Internet is your friend while you're on bed rest.

Don't Be Afraid to Ask for Help

If you are usually the one in your house cooking dinner, doing the laundry and grocery shopping, and running all the errands, you have to get backup for these tasks. Who will take on these duties? Will it be your spouse? Your mom? Your neighbor? Call on help and assign specific jobs to everyone.

Stick to a Schedule

The days will drag on forever if you don't plan them out, but if you know that today you have to pay bills online, read thirty pages of a novel, eat lunch, fill in two stories in your twins' baby book, lotion yourself down, watch an episode of your favorite TV show, have a snack, write your thank-you notes, and search the Web for baby announcements, your day will go by much quicker and you'll feel so much more accomplished once it's over.

CHAPTER 3

make room for babies

....

NOW THAT YOU'VE STARTED TO COME TO TERMS WITH THE FACT that you have two babies on the way, it's time to start getting serious about getting the rest of your life ready. Whether these are your first or your third set of twins (hey, it happens!), you are going to need to make some practical adjustments to your living space, and prepare for the changes in your family dynamic, too.

From nursery design to talking to siblings about the big changes ahead, this chapter will walk you through how to ready your family, home, and even pets for the duo who will be arriving soon!

Siblings' Survival

Entire books have been written about how to prepare an older sibling for the arrival of a new baby, and the birth of twins can be even more difficult for an older child. It's completely normal for a child to become jealous when his parents have twins. The first child has basked in the spotlight for his or her first few years, and then suddenly not one but two adorable little critters come along and rip that spotlight away. Sibling rivalry and acting out are the natural results, but it doesn't have to be so bad.

Since my twins are my only children, I can't say that I've experienced this firsthand, but I've been right there beside hundreds of our Twiniversity moms and dads as their older children threw impressive tantrums, regressed, and threatened to run away if the twins weren't immediately returned to the hospital. Here's what I've learned along the way.

Two (More) Under Two

If your older child is still something of a baby, there is no need to make a big deal out of a new sibling. Kids under two shouldn't feel the impact of the twinnies as much since they just arrived in the world themselves. A few stories about older siblings and extra hugs and kisses to reassure them of their place in your family and your heart should do the trick. Of course, some young ones could benefit from any of the tips below. Take a look and choose the ones that you think your toddler is ready for. (**Note:** If you have three under three, there should be a special award for you each Mother's Day! My hat is off to you!)

Older Siblings

Kids who are older will recognize how much their lives have changed once the twins arrive, and are mature enough to understand the source of all this change, and so they are more likely to have trouble adjusting to their new role as older sibling to not one, but two babies. Here are my top ten tips for making your full house a happy one.

1. Include older children during ultrasounds. If they can't make it because of their school schedule, take a video of the sonograms so that they can see their special little siblings before they even get here.
2. Take them shopping. Let big bro or sis pick out the twins' sheets, swings, toys, et cetera (or let them choose between two that you've already preapproved if you're worried about their taste). Older sisters especially love being involved in this fun chore.

3. Check to see if your local hospital has sibling prep classes. This may seem like a big-time commitment to add to your already busy life, but it will be worth it to spend this special time with your first child getting ready for the twins together.

4. Find a set of twin dolls for your older children to play with. American Girl and Little Mommy both have amazing sets of twin dolls. You can even get your miniature "mommy" or "daddy" a double stroller to play with, and later they can push it right alongside yours.

5. Read twin-centric stories. There are so many books on the market now that were created just for your older child. The author Paris Morris has written some amazing books just for this situation. Pick up a copy of *I'm Having Twins* or *My Twins Are Coming Home*. Paris is the big sister of twins and wrote these books when she was a young girl. *I'm Having Twins* even covers bed rest, which is unique to see in a children's book. I think it's comforting for children to begin learning about this since so many of our twin mamas eventually do end up off their feet. Check out www.myfriendparis.com, which also has some great coloring pages for your older tot.

6. Visiting another family with twins is always helpful. It's a good way for your child (and you, too) to see what your life will become in a few short weeks or months.

7. Have your child draw a picture for the new babies, get it framed, and hang it proudly on their nursery wall.

8. Bring home a "gift" from the babies after the twins are born but when they are still in the hospital. Most kids like receiving gifts (to put it mildly) and will appreciate this gesture from their new siblings.

9. If your older child comes to the hospital for a visit after the twins are born (check your hospital rules for age restrictions ASAP), be mindful of the way you look. If you appear too tired or traumatized, they might get concerned that the babies "did this to you." I'm not saying that you have to have on a full face of makeup and your best updo, but perhaps just make sure there aren't any bloody spots on you or the bed.

10. Most important, make sure that you set aside time for your older child. Yes, the twins will be overwhelming, but your first child (or children) still needs you as much as ever. If you have any sacred rituals (at bedtime, for example), make sure to keep them going as soon as you're home from the hospital. Even if it's just a few minutes of cuddling before bed, he or she would really miss it and so would you.

Preparing Pets

Now this is something that I can speak about from firsthand experience. Everyone worries about how their pet will react to two babies suddenly coming in and taking over their territory, but if you plan for it and get your animals ready ahead of time, it should be fine. A big mistake that new parents make is spoiling their pets and treating them like only children before the babies arrive, only to change all the rules once the twins are born. Try not to do this. You know that you're having twins now, and the trick is to spend time getting the pets accustomed to what will be their new reality before the babies arrive, so that they don't associate the adjustments with the babies themselves.

Think about the places that you'll most likely be spending quiet time with the babies and make those spots pet-free zones now. If you're planning to breast-feed, make the bed and the couch off-limits now, because (trust me), you won't want your golden retriever jumping on the bed when you're trying to get two tiny infants to latch on. If you have a dog, start to change Fido's routine so that it gradually begins to resemble what his new life will be like when the babies are born. This shouldn't be hard, since you probably won't feel like taking the dog on those five-mile runs anymore as your pregnancy progresses, anyway. When you have two infants at home, a quick trip around the block will be the best your pooch can even hope for, so slow down now and gradually get him used to this change.

Another thing to work on is getting your dog used to walking alongside a stroller. This may sound weird, but push a borrowed empty stroller around while you're walking your dog, or go visit a friend who has a baby and take your dog for walks with them. You want that puppy to get used to walking next to the giant tires so that there is no freaking out during your first outing with the babies. You're also going to want to start washing your dog's paws when it comes inside once those precious little babies start crawling around and licking the floor, so why not start now?

With cats, the big worry is that they will jump into the crib. This is obviously a concern with singletons as well as twins. There used to be this item called a Crib Tent, which prevented cats from jumping into the crib, but they have since been recalled. You just have to be a bit more careful now to make sure the cats aren't in the twins' room when you're not around to supervise. Otherwise, you'll have to get a crib tent from a friend or perhaps on a website like eBay. (No, I'm not recommending you get a crib tent. I'm simply telling you that this was its main use for years, despite what the manufacturer intended.)

When you start to acquire baby gear (which we'll talk about at length later), don't just leave it in the box. Set it up, plug it in, and turn it all on. That means the swing, the bouncy seat, and every other contraption that you're planning to get for those babies. It's one thing for your pet to see all of this new stuff, another thing to see it all moving around and making noise, and quite another thing to see it all going with a baby inside, so eliminate as many variables as you can.

When the babies are born, bring their stuff home from the hospital as soon as possible. Put the blankets, sheets, and little baby hats in all of the twinnies' places—a blanket in the swing, a hat in the bouncy seat, and a onesie in the crib. Then turn the swing on, cross your fingers, and watch how your pet reacts to the scents and sounds.

No matter what, make sure you have a backup plan. My BFF had a dog that was never really a fan of kids, but she assumed that the pup would be different when she had her own. Long story short, she was wrong. Oddly enough, the dog never acted aggressively to the baby, but she did get aggressive with the mom and tried to attack her one night when she went to attend to the baby. Because the new parents had no idea what to do next, the dog spent the night in the bathroom and took a trip to the shelter the next day. We all hope that she was adopted and is spending the rest of her days on a large green farm, but that's just what we hope. My point is, decide now where your pet is going for the short and long term if he or she has to go somewhere quickly.

Nursery Needs

Once your kids and pets are fully prepared for the twins' arrival, it's time to get your house ready! You've obviously already given some thought to where these babies will eat, sleep, and generally live. Babies come with a lot of stuff—from diapers to clothes and cribs to changing tables, not to mention toys and stuffed animals. Like it or not, you will have to devote a significant portion of your home to the babies. Trust me when I say that this is not impossible. My apartment in New York City is a whopping 650 square feet, and we make it work with twins.

Yes, you read that right. I know that some of you have closets twice that big, so stop worrying about giving up all of this space to the babies and start getting everything ready.

The first step is obviously to prepare a nursery for your little ones. The nursery does not have to be huge and ornate, and include discrete reading

Note from Dad: *"I nested. I know it's supposed to be the mother, but for us it was all me. And it extended to after the birth, even. We had a room for them, but it was full of clutter from when we moved into the house (if it didn't have a home, it was in that room). I spent months unpacking it and sorting everything from that room into the house (and everything else in the house, too). Then I painted it a really cool ocean motif. Then I assembled all the furniture, then did all of the child-safety stuff . . . I even unpacked all the diapers and wipes and sorted them into the closet and dresser where they were accessible. (And I sorted by size and color . . . I'm a little OCD.) I basically made sure that anything that was causing her stress was taken care of." —Phil N.*

nooks and play areas like every page of an expensive kids' furniture cata-
log. A small bedroom or former study will do just fine. The most important thing to do is to pick pieces that will grow with your little ones so that
you're not starting over from scratch as they go through each phase of
development. But first, think through the big things you need. Here are a
few tips.

Your Crib or Mine?

It seems like there is a constant discussion going on at Twiniversity about
how many cribs you need for your twins. Some parents say that one crib is
enough, while others say you need two. Some parents say that cribs are not
necessary and that a pack 'n play or cosleeper is all you'll need for a while.
Well, let me set the record straight and tell you that one crib is fine, at
least for the first few months. Your twins will spend a lot of time in close
quarters before they are born, and the one crib will make them feel right at
home. Also, you only have one place to check on them at night since they
will be lying side by side in the same crib. If you have a small space, having
only one crib will be helpful, and you'll save a few extra bucks, which any
twin parent knows is always a plus.

In general, twins might sleep better next to each other at first, but
there is also a very good chance that within the first six months, you may
want them to have their own place. Each family is different and you have
to find what works best for *your* kids. One of your twins may have reflux or
some other medical issue that requires them to sleep on an incline. (**Tip:**
If they do, skip the incline pillow and just prop a thick book under the
mattress.) If this is the case, you'll need to split them up sooner rather than
later. I recommend buying one crib at first but being prepared to purchase
the second one at any time. Another option is to buy two cribs but only
assemble one of them in the beginning. This is an idea for people who like
everything to match. If you buy a wooden crib from a different lot (even if
it's the same make and model), the grains of the wood, color of the stain,
or paint could be slightly different.

If your room does not accommodate two full-size cribs, you could consider a mini-crib. A mini-crib is made just like a full-size crib but has a much smaller footprint. If you have room for both (a full-size and a mini), you can consider that, as well. There really are endless sleeping options, but I always recommend that families choose one arrangement and stick

Top Tips from the Pro

I asked fellow mom of twins, Traci Zeller, of Traci Zeller Designs for her best tips on designing a nursery that will grow with your twins. Here is what she had to say.

Invest in Pieces That Will Last

Save money on the cribs and instead invest in the dressers and nightstands that will furnish your nursery. Your twins will only use their cribs for a maximum of three years, but they can use a dresser or nightstand for decades.

Go Vintage

Buying vintage furniture is a wonderful way to purchase quality products that cost less than new pieces. Painting mismatched pieces the same color can help create a more uniform look. However, please make sure that all vintage items you buy for your babies meet current safety standards and contain no lead paint. Sure, this may sound like a big project, but maybe this is the way that we can involve our other family members in the process. If Grandpa is good at sanding, this is the job for him!

Use Low VOC paint

Zero to low VOC (volatile organic compounds) paint is the healthiest choice for all people and the environment, but especially expectant mothers and young babies. Zero to low VOC paint products can be found at all price points from home improvement retailers to specialty paint stores. High-quality paint, however, will last longer with fewer burnishes and scrapes. Paint that has a sheen is generally considered more washable, but flat paint is easier to touch up.

Skip the Changing Table

If you're crunched for space or managing a tight budget, a dresser can double as a changing station by simply attaching a changing pad. Remember that dressers should be secured to the wall, and babies should not be left unattended at any changing station.

Make the Most of Storage

Create a custom storage system in the nursery closet either by hiring a closet design professional or taking advantage of do-it-yourself services at home improvement retailers or organization stores. Adjustable-height shelving and rods will enable you to fit more clothes, toys, and other sup-plies in a limited space. Using baskets on shelves could eliminate the need for a dresser.

Be Careful With Color

Choose the nursery's color scheme wisely. Invest in pieces such as cus-tom drapery in neutral colors so they work with a variety of colors. You can buy less expensive accents in bright colors to customize your look. For boy/girl twins, I often work with colors like unisex turquoise and apple green, because they look "baby" but are sophisticated enough for older children.

with it. In other words, don't move from a crib to a Moses basket to a Pack 'n Play. If your babies get used to sleeping in a Moses basket, it may be upsetting to them if you put them in a crib. The fewer transitions, the better.

Make Room in Other Rooms

Once the nursery is set up, go through each room and every closet in your house and clear out some space for baby stuff. Think about it this

From the MOM Squad: *"Enjoy the time you have while they are on the inside (of your body)! If you have a spouse, go out and do everything that you two normally do and try to get it all out of the way because you will find it very difficult to do the 'couple' things you both enjoyed once the twins arrive." —Cindy B.*

way—what a great excuse to do some long-overdue cleaning, right? I'm sure you'll find plenty of things that you won't miss if you give them away or donate them, so make it your goal to empty one drawer for the twins in every room and one shelf in each closet. Here's how it will all break down:

In the kitchen, you'll need a cabinet or drawer for bottles, formula, breast-milk storage bags, and before long, baby spoons, bowls, sippy cups, and baby food. Keep bath supplies in here if you are planning to use your kitchen sink as a tub. In the bathroom, you'll need space for a baby bath-tub, baby shampoo, washcloths, and bath toys that I promise will somehow multiply when you're not looking. In the linen closet, you'll need baby blankets, baby towels, extra sheets for the crib, extra changing pad covers, burp cloths, and washcloths. In the main living areas (family room, living room), you'll need space for a play yard, bouncy seats, swing, toys, and books.

In every single room of the house you'll need space for toys, books, burp cloths, blankets, diapers, and wipes. Trust me that you won't want to carry your twins across the house every time one of them needs a diaper change. If you're completely overwhelmed by the thought of organizing all of this new stuff, don't be shy about hiring a professional organizer. Even just one session with an organizer can give you some great tips that will more than pay for themselves in the form of your sanity.

Foolproof Baby-Proofing

Many parents wait to baby-proof their homes until their children are mobile, but I highly suggest that you take some time before the babies are born to get this done. Sure, for the first several weeks, your babies will stay exactly where you put them. They won't be able to crawl or roll or move around very much at all. You can set them down on the couch and walk away, knowing that they can't go anywhere, *but you should never, ever do this!* First of all, you'll never know when your baby is about to learn to roll over until he or she does it for the first time. Yesterday, he couldn't roll off the couch, but maybe he can today. Why risk it? Take care of baby-proofing now when you have the time, and then you can rest easy. Munchkin and Safety 1st make a large variety of baby-proofing items. If you can't find any at your local stores, visit their websites. Here are a few more quick tips to simplify baby-proofing.

Get Down on Their Level

The best way to see what needs to be moved or secured is to get down on your hands and knees and look at your house from your babies' perspective. Remember that they will want to get their hands on anything that they are not supposed to have, so move any safety hazards to a higher level.

Assume Nothing Is Safe

Start with the general assumption that everything is the opposite of safe and go from there. Examine the items in your home with new eyes and try to imagine how your babies could hurt themselves with each object. I don't mean to sound overly dark or threatening here, but it's a good idea to err on the side of caution.

Do the Toilet Paper Test

As a general rule, babies can choke on any object that can fit through a roll of toilet paper. Move any objects this size out of reach and inspect any new toys carefully. If you receive a toy with small parts as a gift, your twins should not play with it until they are at least five years old or the recommended age on the package. It's also a good idea to vacuum often to pick up any small items accidentally left on your floor, and to visually inspect the ground before putting your twinnies down.

Bolt Bookshelves

Before long, your twins will be grabbing on to bookshelves to pull themselves up. Bolt heavy bookshelves, dressers, and other furniture to the wall so that they cannot possibly topple onto your babies. Check for loose shelves, too.

Secure Cables

These dangly wires are like catnip to crawling babies, so invest in some heavy electrical tape or a cable organizer and secure all wires out of your babies' reach. Your house will look a lot less cluttered as a result, too.

Plug Up Outlets

Classic baby-proofing items like outlet plugs exist for a reason. Tiny hands love to stick tiny things into tiny holes. This is a recipe for disaster. Plug up any outlets that are near the ground where your babies can reach.

Watch the Burner Knobs!

It may seem like your babies aren't tall enough to reach the burners on your stove, but they'll be there before you know it, so you'll want to take care of this before it's too late. You can buy covers for burner knobs, but many parents prefer to just remove the knobs entirely when they're not cooking.

Store Toxic Liquids Safely

Cleaning products, alcohol, and even medications can be potentially deadly to your twins. Do more than just putting latches on the liquor and medicine cabinets—move these items to the top shelves where your babies can't possibly get to them.

———————

It may seem like you've got a lot of work to do, but rest assured if you start sooner rather then later, your happy home will be ready for your duo's arrival in no time. If it's too overwhelming, plan a family/friend meeting and discuss who can help with what tasks. If you are lucky, you'll have a friend or family member who would be willing to go on "safety patrol" and find all the pitfalls in your home. When in doubt, hire a professional. The International Association for Child Safety (http://www.iafcs.org/) can point you in the direction of a pro in your neck of the woods.

CHAPTER 4

we're gonna be broke!

···

IN ALL OF THE CLASSES THAT I'VE TAUGHT FOR EXPECTANT PARENTS OF twins, not once has anyone said, "We are completely financially secure and ready for the financial impact of having twins." Unless your last name is Rockefeller, odds are that you're not prepared for the huge financial demands that these two little kids are born with. In fact, the vast majority of the expectant twin parents I meet tell me that their greatest worry about having twins is how much they will ultimately cost.

While I can't inflate your bank account myself (I have twins, too, remember?), I *can* give you my best advice for how to meet your family's expenses while making the fewest sacrifices, foolproof tips on how to save for a rainy day while making ends meet, and cover superfun topics like wills and life insurance to make sure that your twins will be cared for no matter what. Take a deep breath and remember that with a few coupons and shifted priorities, you will figure out how to make it work. Now let's get busy saving money!

Your Family Business Plan

Whether you previously watched every dollar or your finances were a bit more haphazard, it's time for you to get serious about coming up with and sticking to a budget. Depending on your circumstances, this doesn't mean that you'll necessarily have to start cutting indulgences and living like a college student. Rather, living on a budget is a smart and necessary way of knowing how much money is coming in, how much is going out, and exactly where it is going. This is information that you absolutely must have if you are expecting twins! You are now responsible for two human beings and the least you could do is to inform yourself about your current finances.

It won't be the hottest date you've ever had (at least I hope not), but plan on spending a few weeknights or weekend days with your sweetie breaking down your finances. First, tally up exactly how much income you each make each month. Next, go through your typical expenses—from predictable things like mortgage or rent, utilities, car, and credit cards to less reliable expenses like eating out, birthday presents, and vacations. Use a few months' worth of bank statements to help you get a really clear picture of where your money goes when it leaves your hands.

If you find that you have a surplus each month, congratulations. You can start using this extra cash to save up for the big and little expenses that will start to crop up after the twins are born (more on that later). If, however, you find that you are going into the red each month, it's time to make some changes. Living beyond your means isn't unusual, but it's not a good idea. If you're going further and further into credit card debt each month, it will be that much harder for you to save for your children's future. I don't want to scare you, but I do want you to stop spending and start saving—now. Think about your biggest expenses—your home, car, and possibly travel. Is it possible for you to downsize? Can you go on a baby moon to the Jersey Shore instead of Bali? Is commuting by bus or train an option so that you can sell or stop leasing one of your cars?

Next, go through your other expenses and take a look at what you can cut. Stop eating out. Start making coffee at home each morning instead of stopping at Starbucks on the way to work. If public transportation isn't an option, think about carpooling to save gas money. If you take a good, hard look at what you really need versus all of the things you want, I'm pretty sure that you'll find a lot of little things you can cut that will add up to big savings in the long run. It might be tough at first to make these sacrifices, but if you look at them in terms of what you're saving rather than what you're missing out on, it will hurt a little less. And enjoying your babies without the constant financial stress of going further into debt each month will be well worth it.

Saving on the Small Stuff

The cost of diapers, wipes, clothes, gear, and baby food times two really adds up fast. Your monthly expenses are going to go up dramatically once the twins are born, but there are easy ways to offset this and keep costs down. Here are my top tips for saving on your twins' daily needs.

Stock Up

One of the biggest mistakes that new parents make is running out of supplies. I know this doesn't sound like a big deal because you can always run to the store for a pack of diapers, but that will cost you a boatload of money since you aren't buying in bulk. Plus, you'll soon discover that it's very inefficient. You won't have a lot of time to make extra store runs once the babies arrive. Most important, stocking up on things like diapers and wipes will save you quite a bit of cash. I recommend that all twin parents sign up for websites like Diapers.com and check out the prices on Amazon. You can't beat the convenience of online shopping, and these sites will ship diapers to you quickly and sometimes for free. Another great source for stocking up is Costco, BJ's, or Sam's Club, which have great diapers at even better prices. They don't have the convenience factor of Amazon, though. I'd say that if you already go to a wholesale club as part of your routine, that's where you should get your diapers and wipes, but don't start a membership just for that.

Now, what exactly do I mean by stocking up? You'll need a minimum of 150 diapers a week. Don't worry—that's not really how many you're going to use. This number includes what's in your diaper bag and the diapers you'll keep in the living room and in the babies' room. You should try to have 150 diapers in the house at all times. As for wipes, you can never have too many. Buy way more than you think you'll ever need. You're not just going to use them for diaper changes. Eventually, you'll use them as napkins, to wipe your twins' faces, to wash your hands, and probably to clean your dining room table from time to time.

Master Sizes

If your friends and family are kind enough to bring you diapers when the twins are born, ask them to bring you multiple sizes! The last thing you want is a stockpile of Size 1s that will be outgrown and wasted. When stocking up on diapers, always err on the side that are a size up from what the twins are currently wearing, because you know the babies will eventually grow into them. Similar rules apply when it comes to your twins' clothing. You will undoubtedly receive tons of baby clothes as gifts either at your shower or once the twins are born. If the season is off or the size doesn't match what they are currently wearing, return anything and everything that you can! You have no idea how quickly or slowly your babies will grow, and next season's wardrobe in a six-month size might end up being completely wasted. Credit at the stores where this loot was all purchased, however, will always be in season!

Rein in Returns

Do yourself a favor and learn the return policies of your local stores now. In most cases, you cannot return diapers to the store if the box is open. (This is another reason to buy and ask for diapers a size up.) Some stores will accept diaper returns without a receipt as long as the box is sealed and they carry the item, so if somebody buys you a case of Pampers and you decide that you want to just get the drugstore credit, you might be able to do that even if that's not where they were purchased. You didn't hear it from me.

Swap and Save

Organize a toy swap with other local moms once every few months. You just bring some gently used toys that are no longer your twins' favorites and you'll come home with a bag full of free toys. In fact, toys and even clothes are items that you shouldn't budget much for. You'll get tons as gifts and hand-me-downs, and you don't need twice as many for the two babies— they can share (unless you're having boy/girl twins and your husband isn't okay with the boy sharing his sister's pink onesies)! If you play your cards right and have lots of friends with babies just a bit older than yours, you might get away with spending almost nothing on toys and clothes for your twins' entire first year.

BOGO (Buy One, Get One—Just Like Your Pregnancy!)

Shopping the sales and using coupons can sometimes cut your grocery bill in half. Before even heading to the store, check the websites of your local grocery stores and plan your weekly dinners based on what's on sale. This is a good time to check for online coupons, too. In addition to the store sites, look for coupons on Coupon Network and Coupons.com. Double (or triple!) your savings by combining BOGO offers, store coupons, and vendor coupons.

Saving for the Big Stuff

College Ain't Cheap

By the time your twins are in college, you'll pay a small fortune for their tuition. Have you ever heard of the cost of attending Yale going down? Yeah, me neither. Saving for college is a main concern for any family with children. Starting small and placing your money in the right type of funds will eventually help you cover this enormous expense. Now (yes, now) is the time to reach out to your local financial provider and see how your family can best save. Even if it's only a few dollars a week, it will add up fast if it's invested properly.

Set up 529 plans for each child and make annual contributions to both funds. Find out the maximum you can contribute per child from each parent to avoid gift tax, but if you or another family member is in the position to do so, these plans can be front-loaded with five years' worth of gifts from each donor. The sooner you fund the plans, the faster the money grows, and it is all tax-free when withdrawn if used to pay for higher education expenses. Do your homework before opening an account, though—some states' plans have better investments than others.

What About the Wedding(s)?

No, you can't think this far in advance right now, but I assure you that it will happen before you know it. If you are lucky enough to have twin daughters, let's hope they choose to marry members of the Trump family! Traditionally, the bride's family pays for the wedding. Maybe you'll end up having a double wedding when your twins marry twins and you only have to pay for one wedding, but no matter what, this is a big expense that might sneak up on you before you've managed to earn the necessary extra cash.

Besides college and weddings, you'll have cars to pay for, prom dresses, tuxedos, ballet lessons, football gear, and all the other accessories that come with having two kids at once. It's easy to say, "My kids will have to pay for their own XYZ like I did growing up," but once you lay eyes on them, you'll want to give them the world! Many families with twins find that it's very hard to save for a rainy day, let alone for college tuition and weddings, but you should always have a few months' worth of expenses in the bank in case a big-ticket necessity comes up, you or your spouse is out of work, or you have some other unforeseen expense. Add college and wedding savings on top of that and many twin parents don't know where to start! The truth is that there are some very easy ways to save up for these big expenses other than just putting money aside each week. Surprise—saving money can be easy! Here are a few tips to make it so.

Shop Around (for Everything)

It's amazing how much money you can save by just making a few phone calls. Calling the competitors of your health insurance, car insurance, and life insurance companies can end up saving you hundreds and even thousands of dollars over time. Open your mind and also think about comparison shopping for everything from gas to water, electricity, cable, cell phone, and Internet. Call around and find out who has a better deal. I just recently called my cable provider to find out about a new service they were providing in my area, and when the phone call was done I had moved my home phone, Internet, and cable over to the same company and saved over $130 a month!

Free Yourself of Extra Fees

Take a good, long look at your next bank statement. Are you getting hit with checking fees? ATM fees? Perhaps it is time to consider a different financial institution. Some banks charge monthly fees just to hold your money. What's the deal with that? Instead of paying them, I'm sure you can find another bank that is willing to give you free checking and perhaps even some interest on what you've got in there. Many banks today are even offering a cash incentive for opening an account with them. Much better than the free toaster of the old days!

Research a Refinance

If you are a homeowner, call your mortgage broker and see what options you have regarding refinancing. Don't forget that sometimes with all of the fees associated with refinancing, it can take years to start seeing the savings. Be cautious and make sure that you have a good financial guru in your corner to steer you through it.

Pay It Off

If it's at all possible, try to pay off any credit card debt that you have now. If that means skipping meals out, manicures, and even HBO (heaven forbid!), do it. The fees associated with credit card interest can spike upward of almost 28 percent. Even if your balance is as low as three hundred dollars, you can save a ton of money by just paying it off. Sit down and evaluate your weekly/monthly expenses and see what you can trim off right now.

Hide It Under a Mattress

Okay, maybe not literally, but sometimes folks have an easier time hoarding cash than putting a bit aside from their checking account. Even if you walked by your local coffee shop and put the $3.95 in a jar that you usually pay for your venti quad decaf skim no-whip mocha, you would save more than four hundred dollars a year! Hide it in a safe in your home or in your underwear drawer. It doesn't matter where; just save it. How awesome will it be when you realize how much you can save by just cutting a few simple costs?

Establish an Emergency Fund

As a general rule, you should put away three months' worth of living expenses if both you and your spouse are working, and six months' worth of living expenses if only one spouse is working. This will protect you from a sudden change in employment.

Contribute the Max

If at all possible, contribute the maximum amount to your employer's 401(k) plan or other deferred comp plans. If your cash flow is so tight that you cannot do this, then at bare minimum find a way to contribute the max amount that your employer will match if your company has such a policy.

Open an IRA

You and your spouse should each make annual Roth IRA contributions. You simply cannot beat the tax-free growth of a Roth IRA, and an added bonus is the fact that there are no required minimum distributions for the owner or the spouse who inherits it.

> **Note from Dad:** *"Anyone who claims they have prepared adequately for the birth of even one baby is sort of in denial of reality. With twins, there comes a point where the two of you look at each other and say, 'This is the best we can do,' and then just do it. Emergencies occur, things happen that are completely unplanned, and one has to adjust constantly. It has been my experience that the very moment you say, 'I'm ready' is when God or whatever powers-that-be ruling the Universe look down and say, 'Oh yeah? Guess what? Here's something you didn't think of....'"* —Sean T.

Estate Planning

Even if your most valuable possession is a wilted old houseplant, you still need to plan your estate as if you were the Earl of Downton. Why? You're a parent now. Wills, living wills, health care proxies, revocable living trusts, and durable power of attorneys are important documents that will ensure that your medical and financial preferences are followed in case you become mentally or physically incapacitated.

All estate plans should include at least a durable power of attorney and a will. The power of attorney manages your property during your lifetime if you become unable to do so. A will is to manage your property after your death, and yes, your twins will count as "property." Your will should include the naming of legal guardians for your children. This is a crucial decision and not an easy one to make, so don't downplay the importance of estate planning. Make an appointment with a financial adviser and make sure that your affairs are in order so that you can spend less time worrying and more time enjoying those yummy babies!

Insurance

Here are the basic kinds of insurance I encourage you to consider.

LIFE INSURANCE

Life insurance coverage is all about determining what you need covered in the event of a sudden tragic death or deaths. Isn't this chapter fun? Since these very well may be your highest-earning years, your biggest threat is the unforeseen death of you or your spouse, which would significantly reduce your family's employment income. Your employer may offer some coverage as a perk and you may be able to buy additional coverage through the group plan. But in general, you'll need more than what your employer offers, and you'll want to shop around to get the best rate.

If you and your spouse are both employed or could continue to work in the event of the death of a spouse, at a minimum you need enough coverage to ensure all your children's needs such as day care and college would be met in the event that a single spouse needed to work full-time. If only one of you has a high earning wage, it becomes more important to have significant coverage on that spouse. At this stage in life, term life insurance coverage is reasonably affordable and you can lock into a fifteen- or twenty-year level term policy to guarantee your premiums won't go up.

PROPERTY, CASUALTY, AND CATASTROPHIC

Before your twins are born, review your homeowner and auto policies and compare them against other carriers for better pricing. You should make sure that replacement cost is reflected accurately and that you are not overinsured or underinsured. Consider increasing your deductibles slightly—you might be surprised by the savings. You should also consider adding a million-dollar umbrella policy to guard against any unforeseen catastrophic losses that could potentially devastate your finances. These policies are relatively inexpensive and offer both protection and peace of mind.

From the MOM Squad: "After the emotional journey of infertility treatment we were excited to learn we were having not one, but two babies. A bit shocked but excited. Two days after that initial ultrasound, we sat down to 'run the numbers.' At that point we both cried out of fear, wondering how we would make this work. Our boys are three months old now. I am staying at home (for the time being) and we are frugal. We use cloth diapers (massive savings), purchase formula at wholesale clubs, use rebate checks, coupon a lot, and buy clothes etc. via consignment. It keeps things reasonable for now, but we are still worried about the financial hurdle of double child care expenses when I return to work." —Christina K.

Top Financial Tips from the Pro

To make sure that your finances are fully covered, I asked financial guru Ann Reilley Gugle, CFP®, CPA, mom of twins, for her top five financial tips for families with twins.

1. Hire a "fee-only" comprehensive financial adviser to help you navigate the financial landscape. He or she should be committed to working with you long-term and understand your whole financial picture. A website like www.napfa.org can help you select a planner who is right for you.

2. Put the proper risk mitigation mechanisms in place. Adequate health and life insurance policies are very important.

3. Establish or update your wills and other estate planning documents. It is critical to name guardians for your children. Make sure that you have conversations with those potential guardians to make sure they are okay with the plan!

4. Understand your current cash flow, project how that cash flow will change once the twins arrive, and plan accordingly. Understand that your lifestyle may have to change dramatically to stay on course in order to maintain your family's financial health going forward.

5. Stay the course. Set financial goals for yourself and stick to them. Remember to build in some "carrots" along the way. Splurge occasionally on that vacation if you have cut back in other areas. Treat yourself and make those memories that will last a lifetime. And if you need that Starbucks latte for your sanity—go for it despite the financial magazines that tell you it's a rip-off. Mental health is a priority, too. Just cut out a few coupons for groceries and that latte is already paid for!

Financial Planning During Pregnancy

Here are a few easy things you can do during your pregnancy that will help protect your finances after your twins arrive.

Flex Your Spending Accounts

If you and/or your spouse has a flex spending account available through your job, max those puppies out. You will almost definitely use the maximum amount and then wish there was more in the account. Some companies have a separate type of flex account specifically for child care, so look into that if you're planning on putting your twins in day care. Normally, you need to experience a "qualifying event" in order to make changes to your accounts. The birth of your children is a qualifying event, but changing the amount in your flex account is literally the last thing that you're going to want to deal with right after your babies are born, so set this up before the birth if you have an opportunity to do so.

Set Up Automatic Bill Pay

This is so simple and helpful. Set up every one of your bills for an automatic payment of the minimum monthly amount. You don't know exactly when you're going to go into labor or if these babies are going to come early, and the last thing that you're going to want to worry about during that time is getting your bills paid. Just set it all up so that everyone gets just enough to prevent you from getting hit with a finance charge, and you'll be grateful to not be thinking about the electric bill on the day of your children's birth.

Twin Freebies

Like the saying goes, the best things in life are free. Why not get some freebies for your twins? Many companies around the globe offer multiple birth programs or discounts exclusively for houses with twins and more. If you go to our website (www.Twiniversity.com) we have a recently updated list. We are keeping the list online since it is constantly evolving. More and more companies are jumping on the multiple birth bandwagon and offering us special discounts or even free items. We strongly suggest that you assign a friend or family member to the task of applying to all these programs. It can get a bit overwhelming since some companies require you to send a copy of your kiddos' birth certificates. It's a great job for Grandma or Grandpa.

CHAPTER 5

carriages, car seats, and cribs...oh, my!

THIS IS MY FAVORITE PART OF THE BOOK, WHERE I GET TO SPEND your money! I could talk about baby gear all day long. In fact, I do talk about baby gear all day long quite often. It is one of my favorite topics. Most parents become obsessed with baby gear somewhere around the beginning of the second trimester, and parents of twins are no exception. This is definitely the subject that I get asked about the most. Countless expecting parents of twins ask me, "What do we need?" "Do we need two of everything?" and the ultimate billion-dollar bonus question, "What is the best double stroller?"

Lucky for you, my knowledge on this subject is borderline obsessive. I make it my business to become an expert on every new piece of baby gear on the market, especially items that are marketed specifically toward twins. It makes me really mad to see any of my twin parents getting ripped off or spending a lot of money on the wrong piece of equipment.

If your last name was Rockefeller, you'd probably want to buy every item that Babies"R"Us carries, but you really shouldn't do that no matter how much money you have. The truth is that there are some baby items that are simply useless and others that work well for singletons but are not as helpful for twins. Stick with me and I'll lead you toward the best items for your twins at the best bang for your buck. I'll cover what you need, what you think you need (but don't), what you need two of, what you should try to borrow, and the surprising things that you should not even attempt to live without. In case you get overwhelmed, I'll include a full registry list so that you can get everything that you need for your twins without even batting an eye. Always remember that no matter what I recommend, if there is something that you really want and that will make your parenting experience better, then go ahead and buy it! Sometimes you have to splurge on a few special things you really desire.

Strollers

Let's just go ahead and start with the big one—the one piece of baby equipment that keeps expectant parents of twins up at night and should be taken as seriously as the purchase of a new car or home. (Well, almost.) Drumroll, please—the double stroller. First of all, you might be wondering if you really need it. Maybe you're hoping that you can manage with two single strollers strapped together or putting one twin in a carrier and the other in a single stroller. Well, you can get away with these solutions sometimes, but eventually you really will need a double stroller. I'm sorry, but it's true. Just face the facts now so that we can move on, okay?

The good news is that you don't need a double stroller for quite a while. For the first few months of your babies' lives, you can use your twins' infant car seats in an infant car seat carrier like the Snap-N-Go or Joovy Roo instead of a stroller. In case you're not familiar with this fancy device, it is a metal frame with wheels that uses your car seats as the stroller seats. It operates exactly like a typical double stroller with the exception that it doesn't have built-in seats and just uses the car seats for this purpose. This type of stroller is a great option because for the first few months, the babies will fall asleep in their car seats whenever you're out and about, and then you won't have to wake them when you get home by taking them out of

> **TWINIVERSITY TIP**
>
> If you ever buy a used item, register it with the company again, listing your own information. This way, if there is ever a recall, *you* will be notified instead of the previous owner.

them. You simply lift the car seat out of the frame and put it down wherever is convenient and safe. Also, this way, you always have your car seats with you, which are great places to put the babies whenever you're out of the house but somewhere you wouldn't leave them in a stroller (like at a restaurant or a friend's house). The babies can sit in their car seats and be a part of the action and when it's time to go, you just pop them back in.

Keep in mind, though, that this stroller is a great item to buy used or to borrow from a friend because it has a very short shelf life. After just a few months, your babies will be too big for their infant car seats and will need a proper double stroller. So buy a used Snap-N-Go or Joovy Roo on Craigslist or through your local twins club and then sell it a few months later.

Side-by-Side vs. Tandem

The first decision you need to make regarding your double stroller is whether to get a side-by-side or tandem stroller. The tandem strollers have one baby behind the other and the side-by-sides obviously have them next to each other. Before going any further, you need to measure your front door or the door to your building, your elevator, and every other passageway you will need to get through on a regular basis. If a side-by-side stroller simply won't fit, then you'll have to get a tandem.

However, all else being equal, I highly recommend purchasing a side-by-side stroller. Many people are surprised to hear me say this. They say, "Oh, but if we had a tandem stroller, we could fit down the aisle at the drugstore!" First of all, your side-by-side stroller is just as wide as a wheelchair (24–33 inches), so it is the store's responsibility to make the aisles wide enough for you. I used to barrel down the aisles, knocking over all of those Gillette displays, and if anyone said anything to me, I would say, "You're actually violating the Americans with Disabilities Act and that is against federal regulations. Should we go somewhere and discuss that? Do I need to call someone?" They always left me alone after that. (The Americans with Disabilities Act requires a minimum width of 36 inches.)

My reasons for preferring a side-by-side stroller with twins are as follows:

1. First, I will tell you that when you are walking down the street and stop at a traffic light in a tandem stroller, the twin in the front is going to feel light-years away. And when well-meaning (we'll assume) strangers want to pinch his cheeks and feed him his Cheerios, you're going to wish he was closer to you.

2. Second, if you are going to spend a lot of time pushing the stroller in a city like I did here in Manhattan, you're going to have to jack it up on each and every curb. This is much more difficult with the tandem strollers than side-by-sides.

3. Third, the baby in the front is going to know that she's your favorite. There will be no hiding it after that! Everyone wants that front seat, and so the baby in the front is going to get abused by her twin in the rear—think kicking, hair pulling, the works.

4. Next, this is really going to seem petty, but when the twins are older and it's time for them to get in the stroller, if you have a side-by-side double stroller you can literally yell, "Everybody in!" and they can each climb into their own seat. With a tandem, they can't do this as easily. I know this seems really minor and possibly ridiculous, but trust me—when they are old enough to climb into the stroller by themselves, you are really, really going to want them to do something (anything!) on their own.

5. Finally, when they're in a side-by-side stroller, they can also talk to each other, share their snack cups, and generally socialize with each other more, which I also think is nice.

Believe it or not, I'm not trying to talk you out of a tandem stroller. I actually think tandem strollers are great. I'm just a mom who personally used both and found certain benefits to a side-by-side stroller. If you need to purchase a tandem stroller or prefer it over the side-by-side, go for it.

Other Factors to Consider when Stroller Hunting

AIR TIRES

If you plan to walk a lot, it is fairly important that your stroller have air tires, whether it's side-by-side or tandem. First of all, they give the stroller a smoother ride. Second, even identical twins can have a size difference to some extent, so when you push the stroller you might veer to the side of the heavier child. If you have air tires, you can take the stroller to a bike shop and have them adjust the tire pressure so that you're pushing straight. The only downside to air tires is that they increase the overall weight of the stroller.

WEAR AND TEAR

Before choosing pretty colors for your stroller, imagine what it's going to look like down the road. Try very hard to picture two years' worth of crushed Cheerios, drippy Popsicles, spit-up, and spilled milk. Take a good look at the stroller's cleaning instructions and which parts can be removed and cleaned.

YOUR SIZE

Tall moms and dads of twins sometimes have a hard time with strollers that are perfectly fine for more petite parents. My husband and I are both tall (5'10"), and we found the Maclaren to be a bit low. It's a great stroller, but it just didn't work for us. Make sure to give your stroller a good test drive before you buy it!

Best Tandem Strollers

Okay, it's the moment we've all been waiting for! If you choose to buy a tandem, you should definitely go with the Baby Jogger City Select, which can accommodate infant car seats, lets you change the configuration of its seats, and drives like a dream. If you are looking for something more compact, you can try the Britax B-Ready, which isn't considered a tandem but an "in-line" stroller. The B-Ready was the first-ever Twiniversity-approved stroller, meaning that more than 80 percent of the families testing it preferred it over what they were already using. This stroller has a very small footprint, makes the tightest turns, and is only a little larger than a standard single stroller.

Best Side-by-Side Strollers

You have many more options for side-by-side strollers than tandems. A few of my favorites are Bumbleride, StrollAir, Baby Jogger City Mini GT, Britax B-Agile Double, and Valco Tri Mode. You cannot go wrong with any of these strollers. Each has its own unique set of features (like bassinet attachments or a third seat for an older child), colors (purple, scarlet, black), and accessories (rain covers or car seat adapters included) that might make it the best stroller for your family. Here are the benefits of each specific stroller:

I like the Bumbleride because it is eco-minded, made with organic products. I also adore Bumbleride's colors, accessory selection (bassinets), and overall look. You can also get car seat adapters for the latest model.

Meanwhile, the StrollAir is one of the few strollers on the market that was designed by a mom. It has the perfect combination of form and function, and gives parents tons of choice about how the twins can sit. If you get the StrollAir, buy the air tire upgrade if you live in an urban area. You'll thank me for it!

The Baby Jogger City Mini is the best double stroller at a lower price point. Overall, the tires create a very smooth ride, the width is very narrow, the colors pop, and there's a huge shade to hide your twinnies from the sun.

The Britax B-Agile stroller sets a high bar in the market, because it has a great seat width, cleans up in a breeze, and folds in a matter of seconds. There is a huge assortment of accessories, including stroller organizers and amazing rain covers, available.

The Valco Twin Tri Mode is the stroller I used for my own twins. After going through six strollers (yes, I'm not kidding), we came upon

Valco and all my prayers were answered. The air tires and shocks withstood rugged rides on the streets of New York City, and the entire stroller was just an overall workhorse. It was fairly tough to clean, though, but they have made some nice adjustments since then. Keep in mind this stroller is very heavy. It's great for urban dwellers (if you can keep it on a first floor) but not the best choice if you are going to be lifting it in and out of a trunk or up and down stairs.

Single Strollers

Yes, it's another purchase, but it's not a bad idea to buy a single stroller (or two), especially if you can buy one used or get a hand-me-down. It's great to have a single stroller for those times when you can wear one of the babies in a carrier or if you and your spouse are going out with the twins together and can each push a baby. You might want to wait for this until they're big enough to go in umbrella strollers, because umbrellas are far less expensive than the single strollers that are suitable for infants. It might also be worth getting a single car seat carrier for early doctor visits in case you have a child who requires more visits than the twin. You can also use it for early on—put one twin in a carrier and put the other in a single Snap-N-Go.

> **Note from Dad:** *"I'm a big online shopper, so I had a lot of input (when it came to gear). And I specifically looked for reviews from fathers. It's not that I discounted reviews from mothers, but sometimes details important to dads were overlooked by moms. We had one diaper bag that was universally loved by mothers, but the straps were way too short for me to use. So when we went shopping for baby gear I was always sure to do my own tests and give my opinion. If I felt strongly enough about it, I would say, 'If my concern is true, then you're going to end up doing all of this (whatever "this" was), because this gear won't work for me. Are you okay with that?' Fortunately, those were few and far between." —Phil N.*

TWINS +1 STROLLERS

If you are a family that needs seats for three, you have some options (and you also have my undying respect and admiration). If your older child is a steady walker and you would like just a place for them to rest their tiny toes, check out Joovy's Big Caboose. This stroller can accommodate two children (ages three months and up), plus a toddler in the rear in their own individual seat. Another option is the Valco Runabout Twin with the Joey Seat. This stroller is your standard (but wonderful) side-by-side stroller and has an additional seat that hooks on to the front bar of the stroller. There was a recall on this seat once upon a time, so if you are buying a used one, make sure that you get the necessary parts so that it's safe.

Cribs

This is another big-ticket item that most parents spend a good deal of money on. Now, I will say that it's nice to have a crib that can turn into Optimus Prime, but I honestly think that you should go for the cheapest crib they make. There's one at Babies"R"Us right now for $129, and I think the buck just stops there. This probably surprises most of you, so let me explain. First of all, I mean seriously, unless you're getting photographed for *Better Homes and Gardens*, there's really no need to have the best crib in the universe. Plus, at first glance you really can't tell the difference between a cheapo crib and a superexpensive one.

Second, one reason some cribs cost so much is that they'll eventually convert into toddler beds and then into full-size beds. But what most of you don't realize is that by the time your twins are ready for toddler beds, you're going to want to involve them in the process of picking out their beds in order to get them excited about the transition. If you're just basically taking off a side of a crib, that's really nothing special to them.

I also want you to realistically think about what that crib is going to look like in two or three years. It will be covered in stickers, possibly Sharpie, definitely crayon, and probably even bite marks if your twins are chewers. Why would you spend several hundred dollars for something with

> **TWINIVERSITY TIP**
>
> A lot of people are tempted to buy organic mattresses, but the truth is, that there is no such thing as a truly organic mattress. There are always going to be some man-made elements in the mattress. My best tip here is to get a conventional mattress and an organic mattress cover, which will save you money and will really be the best for your baby.

this sad destiny? Just go for the cheaper crib. Every crib on the market today is perfectly safe and you'll get exactly what you need from it.

Crib Accessories

Crib Mattresses

Skimp on the cribs, but don't skimp on the mattresses! Foam mattresses are the way to go, because structurally they are the same as their coil counterparts, but a foam mattress only weighs about seven pounds whereas the coil one weighs a heck of a lot more than that. Trust me, when your crib is on the lowest level and you have to change the crib sheet for the seventeenth time that day, it's really annoying to lift the heavy coil mattress.

Crib Bumpers

As you might know by now, crib bumpers are starting to be banned throughout the United States because they pose a danger to babies. Check your local guidelines. The issue with bumpers is that they are typically made of thick, padded cotton, and your baby could get trapped in the corner and suffocate. My twins didn't use bumpers initially, but my daughter always slept like she had been thrown out of a moving vehicle, and she would get her arm caught in between the slats. She eventually had bruises on her arms and legs and we broke down and got some bumpers.

They do make breathable bumpers, which are a nice option if your babies get their faces stuck against them, because they can still breathe easily thanks to the mesh material. Also, the bumpers collapse, so when the twins are older and step on them, they just smoosh down instead of becoming a "step" like traditional bumpers can. The other nice thing about breathable bumpers is that they provide fantastic pacifier containment. Without them, if your twins use pacifiers, they will fall out of the crib a million times a night. Your babies will wake up crying and you'll have to get up, wash the pacifiers, and throw them back in the crib. This gets old really, really fast.

There is also a product called Wonder Bumpers that attach a small pad to *each* slat of the crib (via zipper). These seem to be the perfect answer for a family who wants to use bumpers but is worried about the danger. They are created by Go Mama Go Designs, and I am very impressed with this new innovation. Check them out!

Sheet Savers

There is a brilliant invention called Sheet Savers, which are basically rectangular pieces of material that go over the crib sheets and attach to the crib slats. You can put two Sheet Savers side by side in one crib and place one baby on each. If one of them spits up or has a poop explosion, you don't have to wake the other one up to change the sheet. You just replace the Sheet Saver that is soiled and you're good to go.

TWINIVERSITY TIP

Try your best to create a baby book for each child. I don't know if any of your families had a baby book for you, but I know that it is a seriously cherished possession of my sister's, while my mother never even finished mine. (Sorry, Mom, I had to tell them the truth.) If you create one for both of the twins to share, they will have to fight over it when they're older, so try to give them each one to cherish. I like the idea of including the front page of the newspaper from the day they were born and maybe a grocery flier. They'll each have a cool time capsule and your twins will love them.

Another option is to create a website from a site like Baby Jellybeans. They have a nice format there so that you can just go in after a doctor's appointment and fill in all the baby's new stats. This way, it's all in the computer and can be shared with relatives, and you can print it out or make a book out of it when you're done. Again, I would create one for each baby so that they each have their own separate book in the end. Snapfish and Shutterfly also have great options available.

The Double Gear You Need

Here are the items that you really do need two of to manage.

Car Seats

Obviously, each of your twins will need his or her own car seat. This is a must for the car, for using with your car seat carrier stroller as we already discussed, and also as a nice additional seat for the babies when you're at home or out and about. If you don't own a car you might be wondering if your twins will even need car seats. Well, they will still need them any time you ride in someone else's car, like when you're visiting your parents or other family members.

Think about the other ways that you get around. Do you take taxis? You can strap infant car seats into most taxis using the seat belts, but it is actually legal (yes, legal) to hold an infant in your lap in a cab. If you have beaucoup buckeroonies, you can take limo services everywhere that have car seats in the cars, but if you have that much money, you can afford to buy two car seats, anyway.

The bottom line is that 99 percent of twin parents need two car seats and you probably fit into this group. I like all of the Britax car seats such as the Chaperone and B-Safe, and I love the Cybex Aton, but there is absolutely nothing wrong with Chicco, Maxi-Cosi, Combi, and others.

> **TWINIVERSITY TIP**
>
> If you are getting a stroller that can hold car seats, make sure you get the correct ones that fit with your stroller! Most car seats can hold infants at 4 pounds (some even less), which is fantastic for twin families.

Bouncy Seats

Bouncy seats are nice for singletons, but they are an absolute must for twins! Not only do you need two bouncy seats but if you live in a big house, you might want to consider having a set of bouncy seats for each floor. The reason this is so important is that bouncy seats are the best place to tandem bottle-feed your twins. I'll talk more about this later, but you'll sit on the floor with a twin in each bouncy seat and you can feed them both at once. Bouncy seats are also great because they're a place for the twins to be secure, entertained, and fed—the trifecta of baby equipment! Some babies will even nap in theirs. Plus, the seats are fairly inexpensive (depending on brand), so they win the parenting prize from me. An alternative to the bouncy seat is the Rock 'n Play from Fisher-Price. It will last longer, because it holds heavier babies! If you can get your hands on used versions of either, they are all pretty easy to clean. You may want to consider a hand-me-down or purchasing these from a consignment store or sale.

> **TWINIVERSITY TIP**
>
> When buying two of the same item, don't get the same pattern. That way you can mix it up during playtime!

High Chairs

You won't use them for a while, but you will eventually need two highchairs because you want to be able to feed your twins at the same time once they're eating solids. For obvious reasons, I really like space-saver high chairs. Fisher-Price makes one that converts from a real standing-up high chair to something that straps on to an actual chair. Graco also makes a really good space-saving high chair. Check them out if this sounds like a good option for you.

You Don't Need Two of Everything

Even though you're expecting two babies, there are some items that you can really get by with only having one.

Baby Swing

Most twin parents love their baby swings and many babies are soothed by them really well for the first few months, but it is pretty unlikely that you will have many opportunities to put both babies in a swing at once. I suggest you get one swing, but it's a good idea to buy one that changes positions, because one baby might like to swing side to side while the other prefers front and back. Several of the Fisher-Price swings rotate so that you have both swinging positions as options. This is another great item to pick up at a consignment shop. However, by all means get two if space and money aren't issues.

ExerSaucer

These are great little baby entertainment centers that will keep your babies occupied for entire minutes at a time once they are old enough (usually around four or five months or when they have very good neck control). Once your twins are old enough, an ExerSaucer is a great place to safely put one twin while you're dealing with the other, so I recommend only getting one. It is great to have, but much like a baby swing, it takes up a lot of floor space, is quite expensive, and is generally a good item for your twins to share. You can always get another one later if it becomes necessary. Truth be told, we ended up getting another one. Our twins *loved* seeing each other at a "standing" level.

Baby Bathtub

Since you should never, ever attempt to bathe both babies at once, there is no reason to have two baby bathtubs. You could even get away with just bathing them in the kitchen sink at first (still one at a time). I always liked bathing the twins in the sink because it forced me to do the dishes. That's the sad truth. Many companies make little slings that fit in the sink for this very reason. They work great when the babies are very little and usually cost less than fifteen dollars. It's literally just a little sling for them to sit on. It dries superquick and is great for small spaces. A traditional baby tub also works wonders. With the large variety of tubs (some that even act as a scale, too), pick one that works best with your space.

Pack 'n Play

Whether you're using a Pack 'n Play for travel, naps, or a play yard, your twins can share one for a good, long while. They make a special twin Pack 'n Play now, but I think that a single one should do you just fine. If your twins can share a crib, they can certainly share a Pack 'n Play. Plus, these things are big, can be quite expensive, and take up a lot of space in your house, so just get one. It's all you need.

> **TWINIVERSITY TIP**
>
> If you are planning on using a Pack 'n Play for an extended period of time, please consider purchasing the additional mattress insert created just for that brand of Pack 'n Play. This will give your babies more support than the foam and board mattress that it comes with.

Baby Monitor

Unless your twins are sleeping in different rooms (which is highly unlikely, at least in the beginning), you obviously need just one baby monitor. When it comes to baby monitors, I do prefer the video ones, because when it's time for sleep training (which we'll talk about later), you'll have some comfort watching your babies and knowing that they're okay. However, if you are someone whose new favorite show is going to be *The Twinnies*, then you should not have a video monitor. The audio ones are just fine and are less expensive for the moms and dads who will not be able to tear themselves away from the precious faces of their babies on the screen. Check out the monitors by Samsung, Summer Infant, and Belkin. They have some great options.

Double Breast-Feeding Pillow

If you are planning on breast-feeding your duo, you should consider getting a double breast-feeding pillow. Boppy pillows work for breast-feeding single babies, but they are not created for twins. With the Boppy, the bulk of that pillow is in the front, but with twins you need the sides to support your twosome, not just the front. A twins' breast-feeding pillow is necessary and will save you a lot of time you would otherwise spend configuring pillows to match the shape that the pillow will provide. Look for twin specific brands like Twin Z or Double Blessings.

Beg, Borrow, or Steal

There are some baby items that are great to have but really only have a very short shelf life, meaning that your baby will outgrow them faster than their price tags really warrant. I highly suggest either buying these items used from a garage sale, Craigslist, or other trusted source, or borrowing them from a friend who has one in storage for her next baby.

Bumbo Seat

These are superconvenient for the extremely short time period between the time when your twins can hold their heads up very well (around three months) and they can sit up on their own (six months), and then they immediately become useless. If you can get one (or even two) free or cheap, they are a great alternative place to feed the babies, but I don't recommend paying for new ones. Keep in mind, there was a major recall of Bumbo seats in the summer of 2012. If you are buying a used one, make sure to check that you have the latest model and that your safety stickers and belts are up to date.

Jumperoo

Babies love these things and it is worth having one to see the enormous smile on their faces when they realize that they can jump up and down all by themselves. However, they are big, costly, and only last until your babies can walk. They're definitely not a necessity, but if you can get a used one and have the space for it, go for it.

Toys/Books

Your twins will likely get bored with their toys very quickly, and a great way to keep them fresh is to borrow from friends and keep trading so that everyone gets new toys and books every few months. This will also be a blessing for you, as I promise that you will get sick of reading the same books five thousand times.

Clothes

Think about borrowing clothes from a friend who is "between" babies or accepting hand-me-downs from anyone who offers. I know you might want to dress your precious bundles in perfectly clean, brand-new designer items, but once you see how quickly you go through onesies with twins, you'll happily settle for used duds.

The Skip-It List

There are a lot of items that may seem like necessities but are actually giant wastes of space and money. Here are some surprising items that your twins don't actually need.

Diaper Pail

These take up a lot of space and, honestly, don't hold enough diapers to make them worthwhile with twins. Plus, I despise the fact that you have to keep buying those expensive refill bags. Instead, every time you have a dirty diaper, you put it in a plastic bag from the grocery store, tie it up, and just throw it in your garbage. If you insist on having a diaper pail, you should know that the Dekor holds the most. Make sure to register for a million of the refill bags along with it so that you won't forget to buy them and then never use it again.

Baby Wipes Warmer

People buy this little contraption that warms up your baby wipes so that the wipe is nice and warm when you wipe your baby's little behind. Not necessary. Room temperature wipes will just have to be good enough for our children (at least my children, anyway!).

Crib Bedding

I'm not talking about sheets; I mean those fancy sets that come with a quilt covered in teddy bears and ballerina outfits. You're never going to use them. You're never going to use the blankets that they come with because you're not supposed to use blankets. You may or may not use the bumpers, depending on what state you live in and your comfort level. You're definitely going to use the crib sheets and you might use the bed skirts, but that's basically it. So are you really going to spend one hundred fifty dollars for a crib sheet and a bed skirt? If somebody buys these for you, immediately exchange them for something like four cases of diapers or a few sets of plain crib sheets.

Glider

I know that you see these in the baby stores and want one in your nursery. You just want to sit in that glider and breast-feed your babies and be awesome. I know. However, you probably will not fit in that glider with two babies because those gliders have arms. Your twin breast-feeding pillow is going to have to sit on top of the arms, and your babies are going to be up to your nostrils. Buy your twin breast-feeding pillow, take it to the store, and see if you fit in the glider. A La-Z-Boy might be more comfortable for you, or else get used to the idea of breast-feeding in bed or on the couch. Sorry, but it's better to know now.

Mobile

Instead of a mobile, I prefer some sort of crib light or activity toy that attaches to the side of the crib. With twins, this is much better than a traditional mobile, because the mobile is likely going to be in the way of one of the babies and every time you bend down to pick up a baby you're going to get hit in the face with giraffes. The activity toy or crib light attached to the side does double duty because it entertains your babies without assaulting you and also provides just a little bit of light for when you need to check on them at night but you don't want to wake the other twin up.

Bottle Warmer

A lot of people have these so that their bottles are always at the perfect temperature, but they take up a lot of real estate on your counter if you do not have a big kitchen. They taught us in the NICU to fill a bowl with hot tap water and put the bottles in there until they were warm enough, and that worked just as well as a fancy bottle warmer.

Baby Food Maker

Instead of a fancy baby food maker, you can buy an immersion blender for fifteen dollars, which works just as well to make your own baby food. The immersion blender will take up a lot less space, and you'll be able to use it down the road to make a variety of new receipes from scratch in all of your free time. Ha!

Registry List

Here's the master list of all the gear you'll need.

Basics

- Diapers
- Baby wipes
- Burp/cloth diapers (12–16)
- Humidifier
- Receiving blankets (6–10)
- Swaddling blankets
- Clothing
- Homecoming outfits
- Bodysuits (10–14)
- Side-snap shirts (8–10)
- Gowns (6)
- Socks (4–6 pairs per baby)
- Hangers
- Coat/bunting
- Pajamas
- Bibs (10–20)

Bath Time

- Washcloths
- Bath toys
- Baby wash/shampoo
- Baby lotion/oil
- Cotton swabs
- Diaper cream/ointment
- Petroleum jelly
- Baby nail clippers
- Brush/comb
- Baby bathtub
- Bathwater thermometer

TWINIVERSITY TIP

As a general rule when shopping for linens and clothing, think in sets of three. For example, with crib sheets: one on the mattress, one in the drawer, one in the laundry. This way, you always have one backup. And yes, I mean three per child.

Sleeping/Nursery

- Cribs
- Crib mattress (foam)
- Crib sheets (6–8)
- Sheet savers (6–8)
- Mattress cover
- Twin cosleeper
- Portable crib
- Portable crib sheets
- Changing table

- Changing table pad
- Changing table pad covers (6)
- Dresser
- Glider/rocking chair (remember, not ideal for breast-feeding twins)
- White noise machine/Sleep Sheep
- Blankets (for later)
- Storage baskets
- Nursery decoration

Safety Gear

- Baby monitor
- Cabinet and door latches
- Safety gates
- Outlet covers

- Digital thermometer
- First aid kit
- Smoke alarm

Transportation

- Infant car seat/carrier
- Infant car seat cover
- Double Snap-N-Go
- Single Snap-N-Go
- 2 single strollers
- Full-size double stroller
- Cup holder for stroller
- Stroller rain cover/netting

- Diaper bag
- Stroller toys
- Car seat toys
- Travel mirror
- Window sunshade
- Sunscreen
- Stroller travel bag
- Baby carrier (1+)

Playtime

- Full-size swing (1)
- Bouncy seats (2)
- Stationary entertainer (1+)
- Crib toys

- Crib light
- Board books
- Baby gym/play mat
- Music/DVDs

Feeding (more on this in chapter 8)

- Breast pump
- Breast pads
- Breast cream (Lansinoh)
- Breast milk containers
- Twin nursing pillow
- Boppy
- Formula
- Baby bottles (8-oz. wide neck; 16–20 bottles if you're doing formula exclusively)
- Dishwasher baskets
- Bottle brush
- High chairs
- Booster seat
- Food processor or immersion blender
- Bottle warmer
- Bottle drying rack
- Bowls and spoons
- Baby food storage containers

Keepsakes

- Baby books
- Thank-you notes/stationery
- Newspaper from birthday
- CD player/dock for music
- Twin photo albums/frames

CHAPTER 6

delivery day and your hospital stay

AS MOTHERS OF TWINS, MOST OF THE TIME WE DON'T HAVE AS much control over our deliveries as singleton mothers do. No, it isn't fair, but it's still a fact. Singleton moms (who don't have other complications) can give birth at home or in an all-natural birthing center. Sometimes, they can even elect to have a C-section and choose their baby's birthday. We don't have as many choices. A home birth is pretty much out of the question for most of us, as are most birthing centers (though neither is strictly impossible). Some obstetricians will not consider allowing you to deliver naturally or even vaginally. Of course this all depends on your situation. But the fact that we don't have as many options doesn't mean that we don't have any choices. These are still our bodies and our babies, and we have the right to ask for the type of birth experience that we want.

Many moms of twins just assume that their doctors will take care of everything and fail to prepare for the reality of birthing twins, but that is a big mistake. The more you know about what to expect, the more power you have over the outcomes for both you and your babies. This chapter will guide you through the big day with tips on everything from what to pack for the hospital to how to talk to your husband while you're in labor. Then I'll help ease your mind about the remainder of your time in the hospital no matter what kind of birth you end up having. With the tips in this chapter, you'll be able to tackle everything from labor pains to the pain of extended NICU stays so that you can finally bring home your precious bundles!

Plan for Anything and Everything

I used to fantasize about having an all-natural water birth with Enya playing and candles flickering in the background. That didn't happen. Yes, I managed to give birth to my twins vaginally, but instead of having a "Kumbaya" experience, I hemorrhaged on the delivery bed and almost ended up going down, down to Chinatown. In retrospect, there wasn't anything that I could have done differently to prevent this outcome, but I do wish that I had kept more power in my own court when it came to the birth of my twins. **Note:** I had preeclampsia and have a genetic blood disorder, so my delivery certainly wasn't "typical." Don't let my story make you nervous.

I'm not saying that your doctor is going to let you have a home birth (or will she?), but I am telling you that you do have choices. You can decide who is at the hospital with you during your labor, for example, and who is going to be allowed to come visit you after the twins are born. If you have an older child (or children), you obviously need to decide who will be taking care of them when you go into labor and for the duration of your hospital stay. In a nutshell, you should have a thorough plan of action for your delivery day, and allow for total flexibility in case things don't go the way you have planned. Even though a deviation from the plan is more than likely, at least you'll have a plan to deviate from rather than starting from scratch in the middle of labor pains.

Let me tell you a little story that will help illustrate my point. My twins came early and fast (five hours after being induced), so we didn't really have time to plan. I went into recovery and the babies were whisked away, and everybody left me. I guess they were with the babies (whatever), but nobody came back to check on me for a few hours. Finally, my husband and sister came and found me. I immediately started looking through the camera at pictures they had taken of the babies. Since I had only seen the babies for a moment before they were taken away to the NICU, this was my first chance to really get a good look at them. Suddenly, I came to a picture of my friend Kelly holding one of the twins.

"Hold on a minute," I said to my husband. "When did Kelly get here?"

"Oh, she's been here for a while," he replied.

Huh? Now, Kelly is a good friend, don't get me wrong. She was kind enough to come see the twins, but there she was on our camera, holding my child *before I did*. But how could I be mad, really? It's not like I had planned ahead and said that only certain people were welcome to visit, or that it was important to me that my husband and I had a chance to bond with our babies before welcoming visitors. The moral of the story is that you and your husband should talk about and plan for these things so that Kelly doesn't end up holding your baby before you do. (Sorry, Kelly.)

In Appendix A, I've included a birth plan for you to use as a guide. If you'd like to, share it with your doctor well before your due date. Ask to keep it in your file and go over it line by line with the doctor if he or she is willing. No matter what you have in your birth plan, you should be willing to roll with what the doctor thinks is best. If a situation should arise where your doc would feel more comfortable with his plan than yours, just hear him out and then make a final decision.

Here are some steps you can take in order to get yourself ready for the labor itself.

Watch and Learn

The Internet can be a great educational tool, and to help yourself imagine the big day, you could consider watching some actual twin births on the Web. Many families choose to film their birth and share it with the world, giving you an opportunity to see all kinds of deliveries—even a few water births. You may think this is a bit "out there" for you, but at times like this when the truth is the best medicine, you'll be grateful for these families. Evaluate what you are watching like you did in science class in high school. You may want to watch them alone so you don't have to worry about what your reaction will be or your partner's reaction. Seeing another mom experience the lows and highs of a birth will really be an enlightening experience.

I wish I could tell you that every delivery is textbook and uncomplicated, but the truth is that the babies hold all the cards. They will make your labor easy or hard for you and will continue this trend throughout their whole lives. You have to trust that your doctor or midwife will make the best choices with you (notice I didn't say for you). If you feel like something is off, or if you feel like pushing in one position over another, speak up! Just prepare yourself mentally to expect the unexpected.

Don't Sweat the Small Stuff

Many moms of twins get very upset that their hospital might require them to deliver in an operating room. No matter what, the health of you and your babies is what is most important. Yeah, it's disappointing, but in the long run, your health care provider is making sure they do what is best for you. Let relatively little things like this slide and focus on having the most positive labor experience possible.

Think about a Doula

A doula does not deliver babies—that's the obstetrician's or midwife's job. Instead, a doula is a support person for the mother in labor who is knowledgeable and experienced when it comes to childbirth. Most laboring women have their husbands as their birth partners, and rightly so, but how many labors has your husband witnessed? Having a doula on hand gives you the experience and wisdom that comes with supporting women through many, many births. A doula will work with you and support you in whatever type of labor you choose. If you like the sound of this, you can look into hiring a birth doula at www.dona.org.

Research Different Birthing Techniques

It would be foolish to choose one technique before the labor, because you really don't know what will work for you until you're in the moment, especially if this is your first labor. You may think that deep breathing will work fine to get you through the contractions, but when those contractions hit, you might need something else. The best thing to do is research several birthing techniques (the Bradley Method, HypnoBirthing, Lamaze, et cetera) so that you have many tools in your arsenal when the time comes. If you are planning to have a drug-free delivery, remember that taking a shower, prenatal massage, using the birthing ball, breathing techniques, and sitting in a warm tub are all fabulous ways to help get you through the pain if your doctor is okay with them.

Research Pain Management

You might not have a choice, but if you do, you should know whether or not you want an epidural or other pain medication during labor. These medications, including epidurals, are widely used, but are not without drawbacks. If you are hoping for a vaginal delivery, for example, you might want to go sans epidural so that you can feel the natural urge to push. (Epidurals numb you from the waist down, making it more difficult to push out two babies!) Personally, I waited hours before getting an epidural. I'm glad I did, because it gave me a chance to experience what labor was like—but, boy, oh boy, was I thankful for my epidural.

Get Good Stories

Seek out women who had a positive birth and labor experience and ask them to tell you about it. People will always volunteer their horror stories, but sometimes hold back on telling you about all of the wonderful things that occurred! Prior to your twins' birth, surround yourself with "glass half full" people. This includes online groups and message boards. If you start reading something online that seems to be heading downhill fast, stop reading and find a story with a more positive spin.

Get a Team in Place

You should have a labor team in place and it should be a team of at least three. Your team should consist of the birth giver, who will be the star of the show. You will be out of commission once the twins are born because you are definitely going to recovery after the birth, no matter what kind of birth you have. (That's another thing to be aware of.) The second member of your team should be your spouse, who should go with the babies immediately after the birth, whether that's to the nursery, the NICU, or somewhere else. Then your third team member will act as a go-between for you and your spouse so that he never has to leave the children. Good candidates for the third person would be a mom or mother-in-law, sister, cousin, or best friend.

Have Your Bags Packed

Well before your twins actually arrive, you need to pack a hospital bag that contains everything you'll need during your labor and after your twins' birth. It's best to pack your bags in your second trimester—you never know if your twins will decide to make an early appearance and you won't want to find yourself having to pack when the moment arrives.

Hospital Bag Packing List

A lot of moms wonder what they'll really need to have with them at the hospital when they go into labor. I'm taking all of the guesswork out of packing for the big day with this exhaustive list of must-haves for the labor itself, as well as after your twins are born.

- Paperwork for the hospital, including preadmission papers, insurance card, recent doctor's visit notes, etc.
- Twiniversity Birth Plan (Appendix A)
- Robe and pajamas (Make sure it's something comfortable!)

- Slippers or flip-flops (Remember, a nonslip bottom is best!)
- Bag for dirty clothes
- Socks (Make sure they are not too tight.)
- Extra pairs of underwear . . . for Dad, too!
- Pillow from home, and bring extra pillowcases (Make sure they aren't white, so the hospital doesn't take 'em!)
- Clips or hair bands
- ChapStick or any other lip moisturizer
- Glasses/cleaning cloth/contacts/contact case/solution
- Cell phone/charger (You may want to consider increasing your minutes for now.)
- Address book
- Snacks (Dried fruit and nuts work best.)
- Notebook and pen
- Post-it notes (In case you have to leave any messages for a doctor or nurse, you can just stick it to their office door!)
- Extra bag to take home goodies from the hospital
- Camera (Take along an extra battery and extra memory card.)
- Toothbrushes for both of you!
- An extra bag to take home your day's loot!
- Nursing bra
- Loose-fitting shirt and pants (Maternity clothes may work best.)
- Personal items (sanitary pads, toiletries, nipple cream, earplugs, etc.)
- Going-home outfits for babies (two each, just in case)

Don't bring:

- Work
- Cash
- Jewelry
- Anything you don't want to risk losing!

> **TWINIVERSITY TIP: CONSIDER THE CORD**
>
> Also make sure that you research cord blood storage well before your due date and decide whether you want to bank your twins' cord blood or donate it. Many families are now opting to save their children's cord blood and tissue. More and more studies are being done on the uses of cord blood. Who knows what it will be able to cure one day? Twiniversity has enjoyed working with Cord Blood Registry (www.cordblood .com). Do your research to find out whether or not this is best for your family. If you are curious you can go to ClinicalTrials.gov to see what stem cell research is currently under way.

Delivery Day

All of the typical birthing books on the planet will not prepare you for the reality of a twin birth. Here is a general breakdown of what you can expect during a planned C-section and vaginal birth.

Scheduled C-Section

You should have your bag packed and be prepared to spend a few days in the hospital. Very rarely will hospitals discharge a new mother post C-section before three days. Check what your insurance will cover beforehand. Maybe you can even get an extra day. You might be wondering why you would want an extra day. Well, it's an opportunity to have more hands on deck while you have access to professional nurses and lactation consultants around the clock. Basically, it buys you time before you have to take care of those twins all by yourself!

First, whenever possible, ask your doctor if you can be the first delivery of the day. That way, if his or her other deliveries take longer than expected, you won't be waiting for hours because of the delay. When you arrive at the hospital, you'll be escorted to your room and hooked up to monitors. They will take your vital signs and the babies' signs as well. This is a good time to remind the staff about your birthing plan, if you have one.

Next, an anesthesiologist will come in to run the line for your epidural. You will be asked to sit up with your legs draped over the side of the bed. They will clean the area, and insert a catheter into your spine, which will administer a steady stream of numbing medication. After the epidural is in, the nurse will run a catheter so you don't have to get up and pee ten times. The catheters have had mixed reviews in our group. While some moms love the fact that they don't have to get up and down a dozen times, others felt limited and wanted more freedom.

Normally, after a short wait your doctor will come in and check on you. Ask any questions you have now, while you have his or her full attention. The staff will give anyone accompanying you a set of scrubs to put on before they begin to escort you into the operating room.

You will be wheeled in and asked to lie down on an operating table. The medical team will begin the hustle and bustle of preparing for your delivery. Don't be surprised to see a large team in place—a team for each baby, your obstetrician, nurses, the anesthesiologist, and sometimes other staff members who want to witness a twin birth, especially if you are delivering in a teaching hospital.

Soon your partner will join the party and you can talk for a bit while they are still prepping. Feel free to ask about everything that is going on. You can ask as many questions as you like. Before long, the staff will place a barrier to create a surgical field where the surgery will take place. A sheet will be placed above your chest. If your spouse wants to see most of the action, he can ask for the barrier to be a little lower. Hospitals can usually accommodate this. Finally, it's showtime and your doctor will come in. You can still ask any questions you have, even during the procedure.

The doctor will start by consulting with the team and will then begin with the incision. He will use both a cauterizing tool and a scalpel. You may smell some burning; this is normal. This is good. The incision will take no time at all, maybe ten minutes at most. Once the doc has reached your uterus, he or she will break your amniotic sac and you may hear a rush of water. The doc will soon go in and grab Baby A and lift him up, and a nurse will suction any remaining amniotic fluid out of the baby's lungs and rub him down to stimulate them. This is when you will hear Baby A's first cry. They will then lift the baby above the curtain so you can get a peek at your new kiddo. Hooray, you're a parent! The doctor will ask if your partner would like to cut the cord and if so, they will be handed a scissor. In a matter of moments, the doctor will go back in and grab Baby B and repeat the same process. Hooray, you're a parent again!

The babies will go off to the side for some tests and evaluations while the doctor still has a few items to take care of like retrieving your cord blood, delivering your placenta, inspecting your uterus, and so on. You won't feel much more than some tugging and pulling here and there. You should not feel any pain at all. If you do, let your doctor know immediately.

Now the fun begins as the doctor begins to close the incision. It may have taken minutes to get the twins out, but it will take some time to get you back in one piece. The doctor will have to staple, stitch, and sometimes even glue you back together layer by layer. Don't rush anybody. Just enjoy the sound of your babies' cries. You'll be hearing them for years to come, but for now it will be music to your ears. As the doc is sewing you back up, the nurses or maybe even your partner will bring the babies over to you so you can see the wonders that you created. After the team has you in one piece, they will dress the incision with bandages, the curtain will be removed, and you will soon be wheeled into a recovery room.

Keep in mind that an emergency C-section might be completely different. Always trust that your doctors will err on the side of caution to make sure that you and the babies are A-OK.

Some moms feel slighted that they didn't have the vaginal delivery that they were dreaming about. If you feel this way, talk it out. Talk to your partner, your doctors, or even the nurses. Know that you are not alone.

We polled our Twiniversity families and the top five things that surprised them during their C-section were:

- How fast it was
- How much less it hurt than previous natural births

- How numb the incision site would still be (for some, years after)
- The shaking from the pain medication
- The razor burn afterward (you are prepped for surgery by getting a free bikini trim)

From the MOM Squad: *"Walk around! After a C-section it really does make a difference to walk around. And don't overdo it; it will only take you longer to recover." —Amy A.*

Recovery rooms are hospital specific. You might be in a room with a dozen other moms, or you may be in a room alone with a nurse right outside your door. Each hospital is different. When you are on your hospital tour, check this out so you know what to expect. Once you are in recovery, rest up. You'll need these moments of peace to relax and heal. Take this time to close your eyes and prepare for the long, amazing day ahead. After your vital signs are steady and you are feeling somewhat like yourself again, you will then be moved to the postpartum floor.

Vaginal Delivery

If you are being induced, your predelivery experience will be very similar to that of a C-section. If you are home and you go into labor naturally, that's a different story. You should be prepared for your delivery anytime after your thirty-fourth week. There is a very good chance you'll go beyond that time, but your uterus will be pretty large by then and labor could kick in sooner than expected.

If you're home and you start feeling contractions, grab a stopwatch or an app on your phone and see how far apart they are. If you are having four or more contractions or even eight in an hour, call your doctor and give him a heads-up. For new parents, you don't want to rush too much because the labor process could take quite some time, but you don't want to drag your heels, either. Usually after you've entered active labor, you still have between eight and twelve hours before the babies are born.

If you are home and your water breaks, immediately call your doctor and head over to the hospital. Your doctor will want to check for any sign of infection because the babies are no longer protected by the amniotic sac. Once you get to the hospital, check in and you will typically be taken right to the labor floor. Remember that all hospitals are different. You will spend some time in this room laboring until you are 10 cm and 100 percent effaced (meaning that your birth canal is ready for showtime and your cervix has thinned, making way for the babies to be born). If you feel anything out of the ordinary, tell your doctor or nurse immediately. Keep a steady line of communication open. This is a good time to refer to your birth plan (Appendix A). If the doctor allows, you may not want to stay hooked up to the monitor so that you can try getting in different positions.

If you want an epidural, this is a good time to get one, but note that your labor may slow down afterward. Once your epidural has kicked in, the doctor or nurse will place a catheter in so you can freely pee without getting up. If you don't opt for an epidural, the doctor may still insist on running an IV line in place to give fluids and/or pain meds when necessary.

Once it is time to push, listen to your doctor and push when he or she tells you to. The doctor will assess whether or not you need an episiotomy. This is a cut that enlarges your vaginal opening, making it easier for the babies to come out. Once Baby A's head is out, the doctor will ask you to pause while they assess the baby and tend to any cord or entanglement issues. Once the doctor gives you the green light, start pushing again, and the baby will be delivered. Directly after the baby is out, you will hear a gush of fluid that was behind him or her. That's normal. The doctor will either hand the baby to a nurse for closer examination or lay the baby upon your chest. The doctor will perhaps ask you to help stimulate the baby by rubbing its back. The baby will still be attached and you may choose for your partner to cut the cord. Hooray, you're a parent!

The doctor will quickly look at your vitals, feel your contractions, check the position of Baby B, and if all is ready, it's time to push again. Labor may slow down after the birth of Baby A. Most doctors are fine with letting Mother Nature take the lead, but if there is an issue of a low heart rate or bleeding on your end, they may try to deliver more quickly. All things being equal, you push again. Baby B is born. Hooray, you are a parent again!

After the babies are both delivered, the show isn't over. You still have to deliver the placenta and may even have to push a bit to get it out. It's amazingly large, considering the size of the babies. You can ask to see it if you like or you can even ask to take it home. After delivering your twins, the doctor may prescribe Pitocin to help your uterus contract faster. These contractions help your uterus get back to its normal size. The babies will be off to the side, if not still lying on your chest. This will all depend on their health and yours.

One thing to keep in mind: babies that are delivered vaginally occasionally come out with cone-shaped heads. If this happens to one or both of your babies, rest assured that there is nothing wrong with them! One baby may spend more time in the birth canal than the other, so you might end up with one cone-head and one normal baby. It's completely fine! Babies' heads are malleable so that they can make their way down the birth canal. The shape will return to normal before long. You may not even notice this if the nurses scoop up the baby and put a hat on him or her to help retain heat.

After delivery, you'll be off to recovery to rest. You just completed the hardest day's work in your life. Congratulations, you're a parent!

Here are some specific tips for you moms who will have babies who are born vaginally.

ICE, ICE, BABY

Keep ice on your private areas for the first twenty-four hours. Ask the nurse for an ice pack while you're in the hospital if she doesn't offer. After a vaginal delivery of your twins, your lady parts will be very swollen and ice will reduce the inflammation and reduce pain.

THE SQUEEGEE IS YOUR FRIEND

If you should have any tearing during a vaginal delivery, I strongly recommend that you use the squeegee bottle as much as possible. What is a squeegee bottle? Well, it's a soft plastic bottle with a plastic top that has tiny spouts at the end. You squeeze the bottle and water gushes out. This is the best method of cleaning yourself after using the toilet for the first several days after delivery. After tearing or stitches, toilet paper will not be your friend. Even urinating may sting. Make sure you take an extra squeegee bottle or two home from the hospital, because they are very hard to find in a pharmacy.

BASK IN A BOPPY

Boppy pillows are not just for babies. After your delivery, you may have some vaginal pain from tearing or stitches, or you may have pain from hemorrhoids. Using the Boppy pillow (or your twin breast-feeding pillow) to sit on will make every chair much more comfortable.

> ### TWINIVERSITY TIP: TAKE YOUR TIME
>
> If you end up having a vaginal delivery, remember that your babies are not punching a clock. They are not in a rush to come out and they don't have to be! A vaginal delivery can take days, and this is fine as long as Mom and babies are not in any danger. Don't let doctors or hospital staff members rush your labor unless there is a medical reason to do so.

General Delivery Day Tips

Whether your twins are born by C-section, vaginal, or a combination of the two (it has been known to happen!), there are some more things you can expect to happen on your big day.

Be Prepared to Draw a Crowd

You'll think that you were the first woman to ever give birth to twins when you see the sheer number of people who show up to witness it no matter if it's a C-section or vaginal delivery. I view this as something that is both positive and negative. It's negative for all the obvious reasons (who wants twenty-five people seeing all that?), but it's positive because there will be twenty-five sets of eyes on everything from your blood pressure to each baby's heart rate, et cetera. To me, that's a good thing. I liked the added security of having so many people there, but if this bothers you, you can have a say! Note on your birth plan (Appendix A) that you only want essential hospital employees in the room. Definitely make this known beforehand.

Know That You'll Likely Be in an Operating Room

Even if you are having a vaginal delivery, in most hospitals you can expect to deliver in an operating room. Many hospitals do this so in the event that your doctor has to deliver your second child via C-section, everything is in place. Honestly, it's the best of both worlds, right?

Hand Over Your Camera

This may seem minor, but when you are in labor and delivery and you are taking pictures, give your camera to a nonessential hospital employee and ask them to take a picture of the four of you together. Otherwise, if you or your spouse is taking pictures, you'll never get one of the whole family. Also, when you're taking pictures, be really mindful of what you're shooting. You'll forget which pictures are sensitive when you start showing them off to friends and family, and some of that stuff should not be made public.

After Delivery

Don't Battle the Bottle

No matter how determined you are to breast-feed, you should be prepared to bottle-feed immediately after the birth if necessary. I'm not saying that this is going to happen, but if the doctor feels that you are not up to the job of nursing after a traumatic birth, it's more important to take care of yourself so that you can be healthy for your children. This doesn't mean that you won't be able to breast-feed. You can request a breast pump in recovery and start to pump as soon as you can to establish your supply. Also, you may have to bottle-feed if your milk is taking a bit longer than expected to come in.

Know Your Contractions Will Continue

No matter what type of delivery you have, keep in mind that your contractions will continue after the babies are born (but they won't be as intense—don't worry!). This is simply your uterus working to get back to its original size. These contractions will continue for several days, and might be strongest when you nurse or pump. Just don't worry and take some Tylenol if you feel uncomfortable.

Placenta Power

I am totally fascinated by the trend to eat your own placenta. I didn't do it, but some research shows it may have strong benefits. I had terrible postpartum depression (more on that later), and if you had told me that eating my placenta would have possibly helped me avoid that whole thing, I would have gotten two slices of rye and gone to town. Only kidding. No, you don't eat it raw (unless you want to), but you can freeze-dry it, grind it, encapsulate it, and take placenta "pills" for weeks after the birth. No pressure, no judgment, but it might be worth looking into if it's something that interests you.

Don't Forget to Eat

As crazy as it sounds, your first postbirth meal is very important. It should be something packed with iron and protein—I'm talking about a giant steak with a side of creamed spinach. Make it good. Don't think for one moment that you have to deal with hospital food! If you don't have a family member who is willing or available to make you your favorite dinner, most hospitals have a binder at the nursing desk with menus for every place that will deliver to that hospital. In some hospitals where you have a C-section, they won't discharge you until you pass gas or have a bowel movement because they want to make sure that everything is working properly. So, Mexican food or a little curry isn't a bad idea.

Getting the Right Room

If your hospital does not have private rooms for new families, you may be thinking about getting one. This is really a financial decision. It's definitely nice to have a private room, especially if you want your spouse to stay in the hospital with you. If your finances do not allow for it and you need to get a shared room, tell them when you're in recovery that you'll wait for a bed by the window if possible. The window side of a shared hospital room is by far better, because you have the whole ledge by the window as seating for visitors, plus you won't be bothered by your roomie getting up and down to go to the bathroom at all hours of the night. It's definitely a little more private. I will tell you unofficially the hospital will probably try to let you have your own room because you'll have two babies being wheeled in and out, but the only way to guarantee it is to book a private room.

Don't Be Shy about Taking Supplies

When they bring you your babies, they will be in these little bassinets with a drawer underneath that is full of diapers, wipes, washcloths, measuring tapes, bulb syringes, and all sorts of other goodies. You are never, ever, *ever*, to send those babies back with anything in that drawer. The hospital throws all of that stuff out if you don't take it, so take it. Bring an empty bag with you to the hospital for this specific purpose. Don't be shy about asking for more, either. You just had twins. You can ask the nurses for an extra pack of diapers or see if they have any extra formula. Chances are, they will be more than happy to hook you up.

Take Your Meds

I don't care if you're someone who can get a root canal without Novocain, you should really take your prescribed medications after delivery. Those meds will help you get out of bed quicker, and the quicker you get out of bed, the sooner you can get out of the hospital and go home with your babies. While we're on the subject, make sure you do get out of bed as soon as possible. Tell your nurse, "As soon as I can, I'd like to get up." If you need help, ask for help. If you need to press the call button seventeen times, do it.

> **Note from Dad:** *"I was very worried about holding my babies for the first time. I only held a single newborn once and I was terrified that I was going to drop her. When my boys were born, I had no choice but to hold both at the same time, and somehow it just felt different. When the babies are yours, a parental gear kicks in and it really feels natural."* —Timothy G.

Bribery Will Get You Everywhere

I'm just saying, a little treat for the nurses, lactation consultant, and any other hospital personnel that you'll be dealing with really can't hurt. These women and men work long, grueling hours, and a little show of appreciation will make their day and motivate them to make your day a little better.

NICU 101

I hope this is not the case, but it is likely that one or both of your babies will end up at the NICU. Don't panic if this happens. The majority of twins are born early and 60 percent of multiple deliveries are premature. Doctors define premature as anything before thirty-six weeks. This is just a medical term, so it is nothing to worry too much about. The vast majority of twins who are born prematurely go on to live completely normal lives. That said, a stay in the NICU is not anyone's goal. It is unpleasant and stressful, but I do have several tips to help you make the most of it. My twins are thriving NICU graduates, and I want to help put your mind at ease when it comes to this very temporary part of your twins' lives.

First of all, you should know that if your babies are in the NICU, you can usually be there for twenty-two hours a day. Check your hospital's rules. It is your place. Normally, the only time you aren't allowed to be there is when the doctor is making rounds, because they don't want you to know anyone else's business. So these two hours a day can serve as scheduled breaks for you to go get something to eat or run home and take a quick shower. If for whatever reason you gave birth at a hospital that is far from your home and need a place to set up shop while your twins are in the NICU, look into the Ronald McDonald House. These temporary homes for parents of children in the hospital are true godsends and can make this whole experience a lot more positive.

Note from Dad: *"It was tough at the beginning. You see families in the maternity ward, holding their babies, having pictures taken, and we need to make plans to head upstairs two floors to visit ours in the NICU, where we couldn't even hold them for a week. It was rough, seeing them with feeding tubes, wires, monitors, beeps, and alarms going off all around. The saving grace was the staff; the nurses and doctors were amazing and really made the experience memorable in the end. We thank God that our twins were there for only two weeks and got healthy quickly, because we saw many babies there who were in bad circumstances and we really felt bad for them. The advice I give is, as hard as those first two weeks or so are, the twins will come out of the NICU in better health than any baby who leaves after the standard three-day stay in maternity. Also, you can chuckle at those parents who didn't have the NICU later on when they are struggling to get their baby on a schedule and yours are 'preprogrammed' from when you left. That is when you get your little internal revenge from seeing them with their babies when your babies were upstairs in incubators. . . ."* —Jeremy L. (twins born at thirty-four weeks)

If both of your twins are in the NICU, the hospital will put them together unless one of them is severely more medically compromised. Yours will likely not be the only twins there. The nurses will probably put yours next to the other twins, and you will get to talk to the other twin parent who might be there just as many hours as you are. Keep in mind that in the NICU, you will probably be assigned a primary nurse. You will be spending a lot of time talking to this person, so if you like one nurse more than another, you can request that she be made your primary nurse. It's not a guarantee, but it doesn't hurt to ask.

One of the silliest mistakes I made was to have an outside pediatrician come in to see our twins while they were in the NICU during the first few days. I hadn't even selected a pediatrician yet because our twins came early, but someone recommended this pediatric practice to come in and see the babies. Days went by and I never even saw this doc, so I complained about it to my favorite NICU nurse, Liz. She told me that we didn't have to have our own pediatrician. While the babies were in the NICU, they could be seen by the hospital's staff pediatrician. We switched over, and I highly, highly suggest that you just use the staff pediatrician to begin with. Not only will you get to see more of the doctor this way, but the staff pediatricians are experts in premature infants and there's really no reason to choose anyone else.

You can bring clothes for your baby in the NICU, but I suggest you do not bring anything white. The hospital staff will just throw everything white in with their own laundry and you'll never see it again. You can bring music, blankets, pictures, and anything else that you want to bring to make your twins feel at home.

Note from Dad: *"Wait till both babies are home from the NICU before starting your paternity leave. While the babies are in the NICU there isn't much you can do. Wait till everyone is home, that will be when you are really needed."* —John D.

The NICU will probably recommend kangaroo care for your preemies, which is skin-to-skin contact. I personally recommend it for everyone, but especially for parents with babies in the NICU. If you feel like you're not bonding with your babies or if you're not producing enough breast milk, just unbutton your shirt and snuggle with your naked babies. (Keep their diapers on to easily avoid an accident just waiting to happen.)

Top Tips from the Pro

Here are the top tips from NICU nurse and twin mom Annie Braley for parents with twins in the NICU.

Take Care of Yourself

Your babies are in the best possible hands. While you should advocate for your babies to the fullest, it does no one any good if you don't get any rest and recuperate. Many moms have had surgery (C-section) to get those babies out. That's major and you *need* to take care of yourself. Go see friends, get sleep (trust me on this one!), go for a walk, read a book, take some time for yourself. Try to be there when the doctors or nurse-practitioners are making rounds.

This way, you can get the updates and care-plan changes firsthand and you can ask any questions. Call your nurses before you leave to come in so you know what to expect, as well as before bedtime. Actually, call any time you feel like you want an update, but please don't call during feeding time!

Be Your Babies' Advocate

You know your babies the best (even though the nurses try their very best and may be a close second), so if you see something that isn't being addressed, say something.

Try to Be There for the Feedings

As soon as you are ready, talk to your nurses so that you can start taking over some of the infant care duties like diapers, feedings, taking temperatures, et cetera. This way, you can learn from the best possible source and not be nervous since the babies are on monitor and the nurses are right there with you!

Keep a Journal

Use this to write down your questions, and don't ever hesitate to ask something even if you have asked before. If you forget the answer, just ask. Really, that's what they're there for—to answer questions and calm your nerves.

TWINIVERSITY TIP: BRING A CAMERA

Leave the camera there and ask the nurses to take pictures of your babies for you. They love catching unexpected shots of sweet moments of the babies, and you will always be so grateful for those pictures if you missed seeing it in person.

Bring a Blanket for the Isolette

Nothing makes the space more cozy and homey for the babies than something from you. Bring some receiving blankets for them to use. Just make sure you take them home to wash regularly.

Include Your Spouse

The NICU journey is stressful. It goes much smoother if you two are a team vs. if one of you is always in the lead. Both of you should be involved and support each other.

Please Be Kind to the Nurses

I know it's strange to have to say this, but some parents use the nurses as an outlet for their anger and fear. Trust me, nurses get that you're scared, angry, and don't want you or your babies to be there. However, please remember that these are the people caring for your babies, so there is no reason to yell and scream at them.

Breast-feeding in the NICU

The good news about being in the NICU is that you will usually have access to a lactation consultant around the clock with minimal waiting. Breast-feeding preemies can be a very challenging task, especially if they haven't gotten the suck/swallow motion down yet. Having a lactation consultant at the ready can make this daunting task much easier.

Note: Most NICUs *will not* have a twins breast-feeding pillow handy, so ask if you can bring one from home. That alone can help make the job a bit more relaxing.

If you are determined to breast-feed, the nurses and staff will do almost anything in their power to get you on a path to success. Even if you aren't producing any milk yet, they can assist you with a supplemental nursing system. A nurse will fill a syringe with formula and tape it high up on your shoulder. They will then attach a small tube to the syringe and tape it down your body. The tube will end at your nipple. The nurses and/or lactation consultant will help you assist your babies to latch on and the supplemental nursing system will provide nourishment while your milk is coming in. This will actually aid in your milk development since your babies will be providing stimulation to your milk glands. Once your milk has come in, if you are experiencing further issues, they can help come up with a plan to make the situation easier. There are always hospital-grade pumps, clean bottles, nipples, and any other feeding equipment you will need at the ready. If you need anything for the babies, never hesitate to ask a staff member.

Postpartum: What to Expect

Now that you've made sure that your babies are going to be taken care of after delivery, you need to do the same for yourself. No matter how healthy or ill your babies are after birth, never forget for one moment that you will never be able to care for them if you do not properly take care of yourself. Your mental and physical health are of utmost importance for the sake of your entire family and especially those babies! Here are some common post-partum concerns of twin moms, ranging from the most trivial to serious.

Serious Sweating

After delivery, one of the scariest things that happened to me was the sweating. I was retaining so much water in my body and my legs were very swollen. (This happens more with moms who experienced some effects from preeclampsia.) After the birth, all that water needed to come out, and instead of peeing it out like you might expect, it all came out in the form of sweat from every pore in my body. Apparently, this is normal, but it never came up whenever I was talking with other moms. Also be warned that night sweats are very common after giving birth. Put the fancy duvet in storage for a few months.

Hair Loss

I will also tell you that your hair is going to fall out. This will happen any-where from three to six months postpartum. The Chinese say that when your baby smiles, you start losing your hair, but this has nothing to do with your baby smiling. It just so happens that babies hit the smiling milestone around the same time that your hormones are getting back to their base-line levels. If it makes you feel any better, you're actually not losing your hair. You're just losing all of the bonus hair that you gained during your pregnancy. Enjoy those luscious locks now!

Diastasis

When we're pregnant with twins, our bellies stretch to the max and our abdominal muscles separate. As we heal, our muscles come back together, but occasionally they do not reconnect properly and you will need physical therapy to correct this. If you don't get it back on track right away, you could be in for major reconstructive surgery, so if you feel any pulling, tell your doctor right away.

Fatigue

You will need to take it easy for quite some time after giving birth to your twins, whether you had a vaginal delivery, C-section, or both. Don't think that you'll have these babies and then go to the gym the next week. Expect it to take a year for your body to get back to normal. Remember that it's taking you nine months to build these babies. Give yourself at least that much time to get back in shape. Do not push it—get your doctor's approval before doing any type of exercise, even the world's gentlest yoga.

Sex after Delivery

After your six-week checkup, your ob-gyn may green-light you for some sexy time. If that's the case, you will definitely want to invest in some good lube. When you feel ready to get back into the saddle, remember that your vagina will not be the same. If you had an episiotomy, you will be structurally different and there will be a bit of a learning curve that you and your partner should be ready for. More on this later in chapter 12!

Postpartum Depression

Postpartum depression (PPD) is really common among mothers of twins because we have higher hormone levels during our pregnancies and it's therefore more difficult for our bodies to adjust after the birth. Up to 85 percent of mothers of multiples suffer from postpartum depression. It's nothing to be ashamed of on anyone's part. It is a simple chemical reaction to your body going from having two babies inside of it to none. Of course, it can become a serious problem if left untreated. Many moms do not recognize the symptoms of postpartum depression in themselves, so it's important that you and your spouse both be on the lookout. The most common symptoms include a lack of interest in the babies or the opposite—an almost obsessive concern for them, as well as feelings of hopelessness and despair. Postpartum depression can occur up to a year after the birth of your twins, because it takes your body that long to return to its baseline.

When my twins were born, I can clearly remember being overwhelmed like any mother of multiples. These feelings didn't get any better as time went on, and they actually got worse, much worse. When the twins were less than a month old and still in the NICU, I can remember saying to my sister, "I have to go. I can't do this." I really wanted to leave the hospital and abandon the babies and my entire family. I was positive that they would all be better off without me. In my heart I believed this to be true. I felt like a total failure. I felt that since I could not hold these babies in my body to term (born at thirty-four weeks on the day), that I was not capable of caring for them, and that they would be better off with another mother.

These feelings got worse and worse. Once the babies got home (Baby A was in the NICU for thirty-one days), things got even harder. I stopped sleeping, I stopped eating, I stopped washing and caring for myself totally. The babies weren't my responsibility . . . they were my obsession. I had them on a militant four-hour feeding schedule and that was what my world revolved around. There was no joy. There was no happiness. There were just a lot of babies and a lot of crying.

My husband took the typical paternity leave after the kids came home from the NICU, but took another ten days when the kids were around two months old. He noticed that I was really not in good shape and that he needed to be there for me. God love him for that. He was right.

Then one day I had what I call my *Memoirs of a Geisha* moment. It was when my husband pushed me out of the house and I went out alone for the first time after the kids were born—to see the movie *Memoirs of a Geisha*. This little time away gave me a minute to clear my head and realize that I wasn't right. I noticed that I had taken a bad turn and that I needed help. I was never "there" for my family. Yes, the kids were safe, clean, and fed, but I had barely any memory of the first three months of their life. I can remember looking at pictures *convinced* that someone had edited me in because I couldn't remember them being taken. I couldn't remember family visits, babies' firsts, and many things that a mom should be there for.

I called my doctor from the street, crying. She was wonderful. She was patient, kind, and understanding. She didn't judge me or make me feel guilty for feeling like I couldn't take it. She explained to me why mothers of multiples have such a hard time and it goes back to those high highs and low lows. My body had crash landed after the birth of the twins and it wasn't able to recover on its own.

Medication was prescribed, and time also healed my wounds. My husband was my rock, and no matter how mad I get at him for not unloading the dishwasher or some other mundane household chore, I think about how without him I might have stayed in that funk for much longer. Thanks, babe. PPD was horrible—maybe the worst time in my life, but once the clouds parted, I was able to breathe and actually enjoy being a mom. If you should experience PPD, reach out to your local twins club, our online forum community, or even me. Really. (Natalie@Twiniversity.com) You are not alone, and we will get you the help that you need in order to get better.

CHAPTER 7

a whole new world

I CANNOT TELL A LIE. THE FIRST FEW MONTHS OF YOUR BABIES' LIVES will not be easy. You will be tired. You will be drained. You will be stressed. You will be severely sleep deprived. You will have to learn *a lot* about caring for two wonderful new humans each day. And meanwhile, you will be on a hormonal roller-coaster ride while recovering from childbirth. There will be many wonderful moments, of course, but they may occur under the haze of sleep deprivation and partial loss of sanity.

So how can you best handle this very brief but equally intense part of your life? How will you do all the daily tasks? How will you make it through without doing serious damage to yourself, the kids, and your spouse? Read on, brave parents, for a look at what to expect, as well as the best tips and techniques for making those whirlwind first weeks a little bit saner.

New Parent No-Nos

The first step toward surviving the first few weeks with twins is to avoid making the top three mistakes made by new parents of twins. If you do nothing else right, you will be way ahead of the game if you do not commit any of the following sins:

Mistake #1—Mixing Up Priorities

Right now, your priorities might be finding the perfect color for the nursery wall and a good Father's Day gift for your dad. When the babies come, the only priorities you should have are to keep those children safe and fed and to keep yourself (reasonably) clean and nourished. That's really it. You should not even attempt to do anything beyond that for at least the first several weeks. Putting pressure on you to attend family gatherings or to keep the house spotless will only burden your unnecessarily and take your attention away from what is really important right now.

Mistake #2—Not Napping

My least favorite saying regarding new babies is, "Sleep when the babies sleep." I absolutely hate that. That's one of my big pet peeves. Of course, you won't sleep when the babies sleep; that's when you'll get stuff done if you have little or no help. Plus, when you have two babies, their sleep might not overlap very much or at all until they're on a schedule (more on that later). The odds of you sleeping when they sleep (except for at night, of course) are pretty much zero.

However, if your sister or mother or best friend or anyone who is willing to be on duty comes over, you should totally take a nap. In fact, you should schedule this in, or else you might find a million other things to do and it will never happen. Ask someone to come over at a certain time, and plan to have them watch the babies while you go lie down. Don't be afraid to go to sleep when your spouse comes home from work, either. During those first several weeks, you might not get much (or any) sleep at night, so get it while the getting is good.

Mistake #3—Losing Perspective

When it's 3 o'clock in the morning and you and your partner are arguing over the crib about who changed a diaper last and it turns into a major blowout, I want you to remember that in the blink of an eye, the twins will be in college and you will be crying that their beds are empty. You won't be able to count the number of times you ask, "When did my babies get so big?" They will grow up. In fact, there's nothing you can do to stop them. I tried to keep mine little, but no matter what, I have to buy them new clothes all the time because they keep growing. It may not seem like it at first, but time will start to fly really, really quickly, and you will look back at those first months as such a special, precious time. Don't forget that you will miss the insanity and the chaos of having two little babies to take care of.

> **From the MOM Squad:** *"Remember to take pictures of how tiny they are. I was so tired and worried about feeding them and them breathing that I forgot to capture those moments that you cannot get back."* —Mary S.

Mistake #4—Not Asking for Help

If you feel overwhelmed, realize that people don't always know you need help unless you ask for it. If you give the word, people will usually be honored to help you.

During those first few weeks and months when you, or your partner, are at home with the babies, you will rely on friends and family to help ease the burden of caring for these two little creatures 24/7. In fact, I'm sorry to tell you this, but you are probably already hindering future help from this crowd without even realizing it. I'd be willing to bet that at least some of your friends, cousins, and coworkers have started saying things like, "I can't wait until the babies are here! I'll come over and help you out—whatever you need—it'll be so much fun!" And when they do, how do you react? If you smile and nod or simply say "thank you," you are totally missing an opportunity. Once those babies arrive, you will completely forget who offered to help, how they wanted to help, and when.

Starting today, you should let people who say this know that you plan on taking them up on their kind offer, and then keep a log of who it was.

You can even think about assigning jobs to these people now, so if Jenny from the office says, "I'd love to help you once the babies are here," tell her, "Okay, I'll put you in charge of three dinners the first week that we're home from the hospital. Sound good? Thanks so much!"

When the time comes, I want you to take advantage of every offer you get. Call on those people who already offered their help at random times. Remember, after the babies are born, the shine will come off the apple really fast. Everyone will want to come by and offer to help for the first few weeks, but then the offers to help will start to dwindle down. So use the help when you can. You'll really regret it if you turn people away and then there's nobody left to offer help once the sleep deprivation catches up with you and you're desperate for a little break. Don't let people off the hook the first time they offer; they might never offer again! If Joe from your church says, "Betty and I would love to come by and help out sometime," tell him, "Great, I'll see you on Tuesday at three." Even fifteen minutes with an extra pair of hands can make a big difference. You can also hire professional help if you need it. I'll talk more about getting the help you need in chapter 10.

Mistake #5—Not Being Honest with Yourself and Your Family and Friends

One huge mistake that nearly all new parents make is allowing people to come over for a visit and to see the new baby. This is an even more dire problem with twins because there's so much more to do. It seems so harmless, doesn't it? Of course your family and friends want to come and see the babies! It's only natural. And you'll have a lovely time all sitting around and getting everyone a cup of coffee while someone holds the babies. The problem is that then your guests will leave and you'll suddenly find yourself completely exhausted from entertaining with two crying babies and having accomplished nothing. You'll have missed your chance to take a shower, take a nap, go for a walk, or ask your friends to clean the kitchen while you nurse in peace.

Repeat this to yourself now—there are no visitors, only helpers. If anyone says, "We want to come over and see the babies," tell them, "Sure, I'd love for you to come and help." Make it clear. Don't be shy. If they still don't get it and anyone dares to show up and casually mention that they could really go for a coffee, you say, "There's a Starbucks around the corner. I'll take a venti white mocha, skim, no whip." You have to be serious about this.

I, too, fell into the pitfall of entertaining guests right after my twins were born. I found myself suddenly playing hostess and my husband would ask me, "Why are you cooking?" Of course, my natural response was, "Because there are people here!" And of course I was even more tired when my guests left and I had no one to help me get through the rest of the night. Eventually, I got over this, but I don't want you to make this same mistake even once. Remember—there are no visitors, only helpers. If they don't understand, they will when they have newborns of their own someday.

Mistake #6—Depending on Everyone *All* of the Time

Another mistake that many new parents make is having too much help from family and friends at once. You only need one extra person to help you. Otherwise, your house will feel too chaotic and you'll have to deal with clashing personalities and all kinds of other nonsense on top of everything else. This goes for friends and sisters, but it also goes for Mom and Dad. Often if your parents live far away, they will say, "We'll be there for as long as you need us!" Well, keep in mind that both of your parents don't really need to help at once, so you'll end up with one grandparent sitting around watching TV or being taken care of by the other grandparent while she also tries to take care of you and the babies.

You're better off with one helper at a time, but for longer periods of help. In other words, having your mom for two weeks and then your dad for two weeks is much better than having them both there for the same two weeks.

This goes for all other friends and family members, too. The whole gang from work will want to come over together and coo at the babies, but you'll get more out of their visits if you split them up individually. Just be honest and tell them that you can't handle more than one visitor at a time right now.

Unequal Photo Ops

When your twins are very young, you may find that you've been taking more pictures of one baby than the other. Usually, this is because that baby is simply awake more, and when the other baby gets up everything gets too busy and chaotic and you forget to take more pictures. Don't let this happen to you! If you take pictures of one baby while the other one is napping, make sure that you at least remember to take one or two shots of the other baby when he or she wakes up.

Another reason for this could be that one baby is much more active than the other. When one baby is in constant motion and the other will sit prettily in front of the camera, you can only guess which one you'll end up with more photos of. This is when a good-quality camera comes in handy. I'm not saying that you have to run out and buy an eight-hundred-dollar professional Canon, but get the best point-and-shoot that money can buy. It won't break the bank and will be a worthwhile investment.

Family and Friends Rules and Tips

Here are some additional tips for making the most of early offers of help.

Make a Chore Chart

Does the dishwasher need unloading? How's the laundry looking these days? If you make a list of chores that need to get done, a family member can simply refer to the chart to see what they can do to help. Generally speaking, your family really does want to help you. They do love you, after all. Give them some guidance on how to help you, and you'll end up really helping yourself. A full chore chart can be found online at Twiniver sity.com

Let Them Help Organize

Family members are great people to help you get you and your home organized. Have them help you set up the nursery or reorganize your closet to fit in all those cute little baby outfits. Let a family member go through your linen closet to make room for those baby washcloths and towels. Heck, have them go through the kitchen cabinets to get rid of all the expired food that you forgot to eat while you were pregnant. Having your home in an organized fashion will make your life much easier.

Don't Hover

If a family member is coming over to give you a break, take a break! If you don't feel comfortable leaving the moment they get there, give them some tips and tricks on how to manage the day and help them get their baby sea legs. Once you feel confident that they have it covered, go take a nap. Go take a bath. Go out and get some time to yourself to just chill and relax. Moments like this are going to be few and far between, so take advantage of them when you can.

Take the Time to Bond with One Baby

When your family or friends come over, tell them to "pick a baby." If you find it challenging to spend time with one child at a time, this is when you can make it happen. You'll see that taking care of one child is exponentially easier than taking care of two. Go to the park with one baby, take a stroll with one baby, or go to the movies with one baby. You can even go visit another friend who has a baby. Just be sure to vary which child you're choosing to spend one-on-one time with.

If you don't live near any close friends or family or are interested in hiring professional help for the first few weeks of your babies' lives, turn to chapter 10 for more about professional caregivers for your twins.

From the MOM Squad: "*Do not overdo it. Let others help with house-work, etc. Try to rest as much as possible. Don't be afraid to have your husband/partner/friend be a gatekeeper. It is okay to tell people that you are resting/the babies are asleep and can you come by tomorrow? Or next week? You will be sleep deprived; it is okay to stay in your pj's for the first week or so!*" —Cherish W.

The All-Important Daily Log

Confusing your babies is a big issue that singleton parents don't ever have to worry about. No, I don't mean that you have two girls and you can't remember which one is Marly and which one is Lila. I mean that you can't remember if it was Marly who peed or Lila who peed. You can't remember which one of them got their vitamins because you gave it to them while the other was sleeping, but—wait—which one was sleeping at that time? This can actually become a big problem in the early weeks when the babies aren't necessarily eating or sleeping at the same time. How will you make sure that they are both fed and changed at appropriate times?

Well, because I love you so much, I have included a foolproof cheat sheet at the end of the book, in Appendix B. It is a daily schedule that you can put on your fridge and fill it in as the day goes on. Make a million and fifteen copies. This is the holy grail for twin parents. Every time you (or someone else) feeds or changes a baby, a baby poops, or a baby pees, you'll write down what happened to which baby and when. This way, you'll make sure that everyone gets exactly what they need. Plus, when one of the babies has an issue and you tell the pediatrician that Lila is consti-pated, you'll know what she ate and drank and what might be causing it. You should bring these records to visits at the pediatrician, too, so that you'll have a directory of your child right there to help you answer all of his questions.

As time goes on, these sheets will help you see your twins' individual patterns. You'll know if they like to drink four ounces in the morning and only two ounces in the afternoon, or if they nurse better on the right breast than the left. This becomes even more important when you're not with the babies all day. If you go out, this chart is how you will know what happened when you finally get home. A lot of day care facilities use systems like this because, of course, they have multiple children to take care of, too. For my twins, I kept these records going for eighteen months. I'm not joking. I still have them.

Coping with Crying and Colic

A lot has been said and written about colic, but most people don't know exactly what colic is. *Webster's* describes colic as "an attack of acute abdominal pain localized in a hollow organ and often caused by spasm, obstruction, or twisting." Because babies can't tell us in words that they are having an attack of acute abdominal pain, they tell us by crying . . . and crying . . . and then crying some more. In fact, the only way to know that your baby has colic is by the amount of crying that he or she does. Some moms feel that reflux and colic go hand in hand, and some doctors say that colic is caused by gas or indigestion. Make sure to call your doctor if you suspect that your baby has colic. He or she might be in medical distress of another kind and it's always best to let your doctor make the call to rule out any other issues.

It's estimated that 20 percent of babies will suffer from colic during their first few months. The good news is that it usually goes away by the third month and experts say that colic has no long-term effects on your baby. The bad news is that if you have one (or two!) babies with colic, you will have to learn to deal with a lot of crying for those first three months. I was "lucky" enough to have one twin who had colic and one who had reflux, so we had a lot of crying in our house. If you are reading this after your twins are born during a colicky episode, know that I feel your pain and that thousands of families all over the world do, too. Here are some of my best tips for easing both your baby's pain and yours.

Swing

Our son was supercolicky and the only thing that soothed him during a colicky episode was putting him in the baby swing with the motion on high. Blowing a *cool* hair dryer near him (not on him) seemed to help, too. Experts believe this is because the white noise reminds babies of being in the womb, where they were really much more comfortable!

Use Gripe Water

Gripe water was first formulated in Europe in 1851 by English nannies. It is made up of natural herbs and spices and brewed into a liquid to help soothe a baby's fragile digestive system. There are many recipes found online for gripe water, or you can easily pick up a bottle at your local drugstore.

Keep 'Em Up

If you suspect that your baby or babies have colic, it's important to keep them upright after each feeding. In our house, we held up my son for twenty minutes after each feeding. We did feed him on an incline (usually in our arms and not in tandem during the very colicky times) but then held him upright afterward. If your arms get tired, place the baby in a carrier on your body after each feeding to keep him upright.

Change Your Routine

If your babies are experiencing colicky episodes, you may want to change up your routine. Try burping them more often, changing which bottle you use (if you are using bottles), or even switching nipples on the bottles. Dr. Brown's makes great bottles that are known to reduce colic. If you're breast-feeding, keep a log of what you are eating and see if you notice any patterns in your babies' comfort level.

Movement Helps

Many parents find that if they rock their children in their arms, put them in a swing, or even take them for a drive, these distractions will help with the crying. Some experts feel that the movement helps ease their digestion and makes them more comfortable.

When All Else Fails, Accept It!

Sometimes, no matter what you do, you just have to accept that your baby or babies have colic. Luckily, it doesn't last forever. My mom told me that I was so colicky that she often dressed me up as if we were going out, put me in my carriage, and then opened all the windows and strolled me around the house when I just wouldn't stop crying. I cried so much that my sister (who was only three years old at the time) can actually remember asking my mom, "Can we just shut this kid up?" Even the most colicky babies can grow into little angels—just look at me! My mother quickly forgave me for all of my colicky sins.

Swaddle Them

Swaddling means basically wrapping them tightly in a blanket, which is said to replicate the womb environment and help babies sleep. To swaddle a baby, take a large blanket (I like Aden + Anais swaddling blankets because they are big and made from a breathable fabric) and fold down the top to form a triangle. Place the baby on the blanket so that only its head is above the line of the blanket. Take the right side of the blanket, wrap it around his body really tightly, and tuck it behind his left arm. Then take the bottom of the blanket and tuck it tightly behind the baby's right arm. Finally, take the left side of the blanket, wrap it around as many times as you can, and then tuck it all in. Don't be afraid to make it really tight! If this is too complicated for you, you can purchase swaddle blankets that attach with Velcro and are basically a cheat sheet.

Co-Swaddling

Some twin parents swear by co-swaddling their twins. This is how to do it safely:

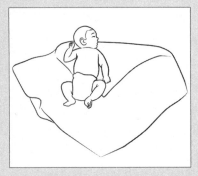

Using a swaddling blanket (not a receiving blanket) like Aden + Anais, simply fold one edge over, forming a large triangle. Place one baby on top of the blanket so that the head is above the fold in the center of the blanket.

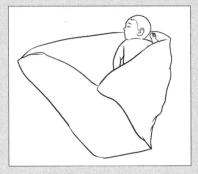

Fold one side of the blanket over and tuck it firmly beneath the baby.

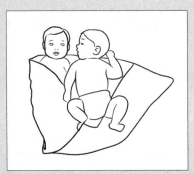

Place the next twinnie next to the baby in mid-swaddle.

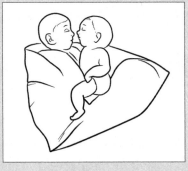

Position second twinnie facing the other. Be mindful to position the baby's hands in a way they like best. Perhaps they like to chew on their hands, or the hands of their twin, so put their hands up near their face (this is optional—this is just how my twinnies liked to be). Be sure their nails are filed down so they don't scratch each other.

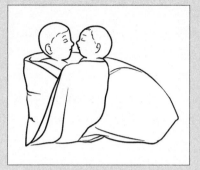

Fold the bottom portion of the swaddling blanket behind the newly added baby. Tuck firmly behind the baby.

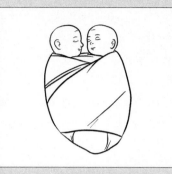

Fold the remaining blanket edge firmly around BOTH babies. Secure the blanket tip by tucking a corner into the swaddle. Be sure both babies are tucked in firmly but not too tight. They should have restricted movement to feel secure (womb-like) and not be able to wiggle free easily but loose enough that it won't interfere with their breathing.

Note: When co-swaddling your twins, be sure to keep an eye on them. You should never leave co-swaddled babies unattended unless otherwise recommended by your health care professional.

Pacifiers 101

While singleton parents can often take pacifiers or leave them, many parents of multiples find that pacifiers are a must-have in their newborns' lives. A pacifier is a great tool to help soothe one child while you tend to the other, and can save your sanity when your twins cry "in stereo." Here are a few additional reasons that parents of twins often can't live without pacifiers.

- They soothe a fussy baby, or two, or three, or four.
- They help your babies fall asleep. (The sucking motion is very soothing to newborns/infants.)

- They provide a distraction while you tend to your other kiddos.
- Pacifiers might reduce the risk of SIDS.
- Pacifiers are disposable. You can give the pacifiers to the "pacifier fairy," but thumb sucking is *much* harder to stop.

If you are interested in introducing pacifiers to your twins, here are some tips for getting the most out of that little binky.

Wait for the Right Time

If you are breast-feeding, wait until your nursing routine is well established and your babies are latching well before introducing a pacifier. Giving a pacifier to your breast-feeding baby too soon (within the first three to four weeks) might interfere with a baby's ability to latch or create "nipple confusion."

Pick the Right One

Make sure to choose the proper pacifier for your twins. Look for one that is made of silicone, all one piece, and dishwasher safe. The latex variety can break down over time, creating a potential choking hazard for your children. MAM makes exceptional pacifiers that have been preferred by Twiniversity families for years.

Keep It Clean

Clean it, clean it, clean it! Using dish soap, a pacifier cleaner, or fresh water can help lessen the germs that your pacifiers carry into your twins' mouths. If you have a sterilizer, throw the pacifiers in with the bottles. Otherwise, think about investing in some micro steam bags. *Never* use your own mouth as a form of cleaning the pacifier.

Replace It Regularly

Check the pacifiers often and replace them at the first sign of wear and tear. This will ensure that they are safe, clean, and the right size for your children.

Pacifier Weaning

If your twins do grow attached to their pacifiers, you may have some anxiety about weaning them. When is it time to get rid of that binky once and for all? Here are some tips about how and when to wean your twins from their pacifiers when the time comes down the road.

Fairy Tales

A popular method is to put the pacifiers in a box and tell your twins that the pacifier fairy is coming to bring them to new babies who need them. When the twins fall asleep, throw out the pacifiers and replace them with a cute present from the pacifier fairy.

Go Cold Turkey

Obviously, you can just get rid of them one day and that'll be it. You can expect some fussing for a few days, but probably not much more.

Swap It

Many parents replace the pacifiers with soft animals to cuddle, or even sew the pacifiers into a stuffed animal to create a special buddy, then just remove the pacifier part but let the animal remain.

Look for an Opportunity

If one or both of your twins has a stuffy nose and needs to sleep without a pacifier for a few nights in order to breathe, simply use this as an opportunity to lose the pacifier altogether. Once the cold is gone, just don't bring the pacifier back. Chances are, now that your little ones know they can sleep without it, they'll do just that.

Diapering Your Duo

Right now you may have no idea how to change a diaper, but trust that just a few days after your twins' birth you will be a pro! As newborns, your twins will go through roughly nine or ten diapers a day each. That's a lot of diapers, a lot of wipes, and a lot of time for you to spend at the changing table. Here are some diapering tips to begin your mastery of this very essential task.

Designate an Area—or Two!

Set up at least one or two designated areas in your house for diaper changes. With all those diapers to change and two babies to look after, you won't want to trudge up and down a flight of stairs for each diaper change. Make sure that each designated diaper change area is stocked with diapers, wipes, and diaper rash cream.

Change before Feedings

It's better to change your babies before feeding them, especially if it's the middle of the night or you're hoping your babies will go to sleep after eating. Of course, you'll run the risk of having to change them again after they eat. Also, if they are fresh and clean, they will eat better!

Sing to Your Babies

Diaper changes don't have to feel like a business transaction! Take the opportunity to sing or talk to your little ones, blow raspberries on their tummies, or snuggle into their necks for some kisses. Even the most mundane moment can be a great time to interact with your babies.

Don't Let Go

Always keep a grip on your baby when he or she is on the changing table to prevent falls. **Note:** If your changing table or changing pad has a strap attached to secure the baby, please use it.

Change One at a Time

Never put two babies on the changing table at once. Change one baby, put him in a safe place like strapped into a bouncy seat or swing, and then change the other baby.

Wipe Front to Back

When changing a girl, always wipe front to back to prevent fecal matter from getting into her vagina. (This can cause infection.)

Don't Bother with Tee Pees

When diapering a boy, simply tuck his penis down to prevent getting showered. Those "pee pee tee pees" aren't really necessary. **Note:** You will get peed on at one time or another. It's one of the great joys of parenthood.

Disposable vs. Cloth Diapers

Despite the green movement that has been picking up steam over the past few years, most moms still use disposable diapers for their twins. But there are pros and cons to both disposable and cloth diapers, and both can be costly. When it comes to disposable diapers, there is no one "best" brand. Different brands fit different babies differently and you will soon develop your own personal preference. Here are some of the pros of disposable diapers:

- They keep your baby drier for longer, resulting in fewer diaper changes throughout the day.
- They require less work from you, and don't need to be washed.
- They are easier to deal with when traveling or just leaving the house.
- They are often less expensive than cloth diapers when the cost of washing is factored in, and you don't need to make a large initial investment as with cloth diapers.

On the other hand, while a lot of moms worry that it is a crazy idea to use cloth diapers on their twins, that's definitely not the case. Cloth diapers have changed a lot since we were babies—they now have snaps or Velcro and come in all sorts of cute designs for your little ones. There are several reasons why many twin mamas prefer using cloth diapers for their twins. Here are some of the biggest pluses to cloth diapers:

- Once you've purchased all of the cloth diapers and liners, you might save money over disposable diapers.
- You can rest assured that you are not destroying the planet by filling our landfills with your twins' dirty diapers.
- They are all natural with no chemicals.
- Babies who wear cloth diapers often potty train earlier, because they are more familiar with their bodily functions.
- Disposable diapers for your twins will cost you more than four thousand dollars compared to around a thousand dollars (not including water) for cloth.

Babies' Bath Time

Bath time for your twins can be one of the best parts of the day and also one of the scariest because of their tiny, slippery, squirmy bodies. Full baths are not necessary every day for your newborns, since they are just sitting around for most of the day and probably aren't getting too dirty. Save the daily scrubs for the sandbox days ahead of you! For the first month or so, baths a few times a week is more than enough—washing them more often can actually dry out your newborns' delicate skin. A sponge bath may be the easiest way to clean your babies when they first come home, but once they've graduated to a real bath, here are some tips to keep in mind.

One Baby at a Time

Unless you have two adults bathing two babies, you should always bathe your twins one at a time for the first few months—until they can sit up really well on their own. Bathing two babies together is very dangerous and should never, ever be done until they get much bigger.

Prep the Area

Once you have a baby in the bath, your complete attention should be focused on him or her, so make sure that you have everything that you need set up beforehand. This includes soap, towels, washcloths, bath toys, et cetera. It's also a good idea to make sure that your hands are free by placing the baby shampoo in a bottle with a pump. Always keep one hand on your baby while she's in the bath.

Check the Temp

A baby's bathwater should be about 97–100 degrees (36–38 C). This is not too hot or too cold. As Goldilocks said, "It's just right!" You can buy rubber duckies that light up if they're placed in water that's too hot for infants, so pick up one of those guys to take the guesswork out of the equation. And most important, don't put a baby in a tub as it is being filled! Running water can change temperature quickly, and can injure your little ones. It takes ten seconds for a baby to get a third-degree burn from water that is 140 degrees, and only five seconds if it is 150 degrees. Start with only two to three inches of water in the tub. Newborns are tiny and don't really need to be submerged in the water. You only need enough to clean them off.

Keep the Room Warm

Babies are little and lose body heat quickly, so make sure that the room you bathe them in is nice and warm, and wrap them in a cute little hooded towel as soon as you get them out of the water. A room temperature of about 75 degrees is ideal for your twinnies.

Save the Dirtiest for Last

Remember to wash your babies' dirtiest parts last! Start off with their faces and work your way down. Don't miss any chubby folds—milk and spit-up love to hide out in these crevices.

Note from Dad: "Anytime I hear a dad of a single child complain about difficulty, I always say to myself, 'If only you had two.' I get pleasure knowing that I am successful in doing something that's twice as hard." —Timothy G.

Bathe Together!

If you have an extra pair of hands nearby, indulge in some fun bonding time by taking the twins in the tub with you—only one at a time, of course. This is a great way to snuggle and get close to your babies, but remember to be safe and save the fancy scented bath oils for another time. **Warning:** Babies are slippery when wet!

Common Infant Health Issues

During your twins' first few weeks at home, you will be in awe of their amazing new bodies, and probably worry about symptoms that are totally normal in newborns—you just never knew about them! Here are some of the most common infant issues and how to best handle them.

Baby Acne

Baby acne usually appears around a baby's one month birthday and sticks around for a few weeks before disappearing. Just like the name implies, baby acne is acne . . . on your babies! It is caused by the mother's hormones that seep into the baby at the end of the pregnancy. While baby acne might make your precious twins a bit less photogenic than normal for a few weeks, it is otherwise completely harmless. Don't bother your babies by applying pimple cream or searching for remedies. Simply ignore baby acne and it will disappear for at least twelve or thirteen years.

Reflux

Baby reflux is just like reflux in adults. It is caused when the valve connecting the esophagus to the stomach doesn't work properly. It is quite common in babies because this system is still developing. Many babies experience reflux during their first few months, only to have it disappear thereafter. Reflux is also more common in premature infants. Signs of reflux in infants include excessive spit-up, gagging during feedings, and other signs of abdominal pain. Many doctors will prescribe medications for reflux, so talk to your pediatrician if you suspect that one or both of your babies may be suffering. **Note:** The Twiniversity website is filled with tips on dealing with reflux. Check them out if necessary.

No Tear Ducts

Newborns' tear ducts aren't fully formed until they are about one year old. And you thought that babies needed tears in order to cry! They'll be able to cry without tears just fine, but your twins might wake up with gooey eyes that are a sign of a clogged tear duct. This is very common. Simply apply a gentle warm compress (like a damp, warm cotton ball) over the area a few times a day and it should clear up on its own. If not, call your pediatrician.

Variable Body Temperature

Newborns aren't able to retain their body temperature, so it's very important that you keep them nice and warm. However, babies also run the risk of becoming overheated for this same reason. A good general rule is to dress your twins in similar clothes to you and then add one additional layer. So if you are sleeping in pajamas, your twins should be sleeping in pajamas and a sleep sack. Keep your home at a warm but comfortable temperature (about 70 degrees) and don't be afraid to snuggle up close to help your babies' bodies reach the proper temperature.

Daily Logistics with Two

Mothers of singletons will never know the juggling act it takes to make it through each day with twin newborns. But we've all lived to tell the tale, and you will, too.

Immediately Outnumbered

The first time you are at home alone with your twins, you'll immediately realize that you are officially outnumbered. Twin babies outnumber mommies two to one—all the time! Don't let this scare you; just plan on having as much help as you can. Always try to look on the bright side—Mother Nature gave you two arms and two legs to hold each baby. You will find a way to manage both babies at once. I strongly advise finding a triplet mom in your local area. She will offer you perspective that you can't find any-place else and make you feel like you have it easy!

But it's true that it will be a very rare moment when you are not using both hands to the fullest. There will be many times when both babies want to be held. Many hours of the day will be spent feeding two babies at once (more on this in chapter 8). When you're out and about, you're always using both hands to push the stroller, wipe drool, reach for a toy, and so on. You'll quickly find that you're more than willing to give up that fashionable handbag for something more functional that goes over your shoulder (or even a backpack-style diaper bag). Function will have to come before form for a while.

Choosing between Babies

There are going to be times when both babies are crying or hungry and want your attention, and you are going to have to choose which baby to tend to first. If one baby always cries louder, it may be tempting to always go to her first, but sometimes the quieter baby needs you just as much. Go with your gut on this one, and you will find a way to soothe them both. This is when those two arms come in handy (see above).

Double Identity

It is very common for new mothers to experience a bit of an identity crisis during the first few weeks at home with a new baby, and as with many things, it is often more exaggerated with twins. Depending on your lifestyle before the babies arrived, your entire universe is probably about to do a complete 180. Even if you are already a mom, having two new babies will rock your world and your sense of self in ways that you probably can't even imagine. This is completely common and normal. During the first few weeks at home with twins, the child care is all encompassing. You spend day and night feeding, changing, and soothing babies. Often, you lose track of what is going on in the rest of the world or the fact that the rest of the world even exists. Soon enough, you begin to wonder who you really are and what has happened to the thing you thought was your life! Well, your life will be yours again one day, but your identity will need to do some serious adjusting in the meantime so that you can begin to view yourself as a mother *and* the person you used to be. Here are some tips for dealing with this identity crisis.

Get Out of the House

It is so tempting to just hunker down and hibernate for the first several weeks of your babies' lives. They aren't supposed to be exposed to germs, it's so much effort to get out in the first place, and weather may be yet another factor keeping you indoors (depending on the season and where you live). Despite all of this, I strongly urge you to get out. Get out with the babies or get out without the babies. It doesn't matter what you do or where you do it—just go outside, walk around the block, get a coffee, or go for a drive. Disengage from the constant caregiving and give yourself a few moments just for you.

Do Things You Used to Enjoy

What were your favorite things to do before having twins? Did you love to go to the movies, read cheesy thrillers, or make scrapbooks for your friends?

I know that you don't have time to do this stuff anymore, but you have to make the time. Read a book for ten minutes before bed or watch a movie on Netflix after the babies are asleep. Use your love of scrapbooking to make the twins a rocking baby book! Continuing with activities that you used to enjoy is key to remembering who you are and who you will continue to be.

Catch Up with Friends

Friends will surely be calling you to ask how you and the babies are doing, and it may be tempting to spend the entire phone call or visit talking about the cute things that they did or how tired you are, but try to spend some time catching up on your friends' lives, too. First of all, it will certainly make you a better friend, but it will also help you remember that there is more to life than diapers and spit-up.

Catch Up on News

Your twins might be your entire world right now, but there *is* a big, beautiful world out there, too. While it may be healthy to take a break from the tabloids and reality shows, try to stay in the loop when it comes to big news. It will help you keep last night's crying jag in perspective.

Dress for Success

Of course it's easier to wear pajama pants and your husband's old T-shirt all day, and there will be a lot of days when that's the best you can manage, and that's fine. But dressing like your old self will help you feel more like your old self. No, you shouldn't wear your most expensive power suit and stilettos to take care of the twins all day, but taking the time to put on real clothes, real shoes, and even some lip gloss will make you feel a bit more human and a lot less like a shut-in.

◎◎

One-on-One Time

I have heard so many mothers of twins shamefully say that they have very few specific memories from their twins' first year. Many of them recall this time period as one huge blur of crying, sleeplessness, endless feedings, and dirty diapers, and they have a visceral memory only of how this time felt physically—the sheer exhaustion, the emotional depletion that comes with being responsible for two babies, and the painful loss of their prepregnancy identity and lifestyle. They feel guilty about not having positive memories of time they actually spent with their babies. While it's very difficult to create lasting memories when you are busy caring for two, you must carve out some one-on-one time with each of your twins to take time for those special moments and strengthen your bond with each one.

Spending time alone with each baby will revitalize your relationship with each of them and increase your ability to connect. Without the other sibling present, you won't feel pulled in two different directions at once. And you can learn to appreciate each baby's distinct temperament and personality. Getting to know both of your children on this level is important for the future emotional well-being of you and your babies.

Enjoying some one-on-one time during your twins' first few months will also help you realize that they can thrive while being separated from each other. Infants are individuals first and twins second, something that is important for all of you to honor throughout their lives. Start putting this perspective into practice early on by bonding with them as individuals.

- Here are some easy and fun things that you can do with your one-on-one twin time. To make the most of these moments and create priceless memories, no texting or talking on the phone is allowed during these activities!
- Cherish bath time when you bathe each of the babies separately— you can't beat this precious bonding time.

- Take one baby out with you for a walk in the single stroller or baby carrier.
- Take each of the twins separately for doctor's appointments.
- Bring them to a play group or new-moms' group on opposite days.
- Play with one baby alone at the park or push one baby in a baby swing at the playground.

Note from Dad: *"Create special times for you and the babies. Take them out every Sunday morning (or something similar)—it doesn't need to be fancy but spend time alone with them."* —Mike B.

Top Tips from the Pro

For more advice about how to deal with the identity issues that may arrive along with your new duo, I asked twin expert (and twin mom) Joan Friedman, PhD, for her top five tips for staying balanced and feeling like yourself. Here are her ideas.

1. Find ways to laugh about anything and everything. Connecting to your sense of humor is an excellent way of reconnecting to yourself.
2. Go shopping, and not just for baby things! If finances are an issue, give yourself a very small budget (say five dollars) to buy one fun little treat for yourself.
3. Have coffee with a friend who does not have children so that you can be reminded of the good and bad aspects of how "the other half lives."
4. Get together with a mentor who is not a family member. He or she will remind you of who you are and what you want in life.

5. Try something new that you didn't do before having babies. If you used to do yoga, try Pilates. This is a way of telling yourself that you really are a different person now and that's okay!

Making Milestones

Here's a general overview of the developmental milestones for newborns in the first year.* You won't believe how fast they'll change! Keep in mind one of the most challenging parts of being a parent of twins is not comparing your children when it comes to developmental milestones (and everything else!). When one of my twins first rolled over, I quickly looked at the other baby to see if that one would roll, too. When one said their first word, I wondered when the other would say theirs. Even though I knew that they were two different people, it was very difficult not to constantly compare them to one another. If you see the gap between their milestones getting bigger, don't hesitate to point it out to your pediatrician, but otherwise don't forget that if they aren't identical, they are simply siblings with the same birthday (and even identical twins aren't exactly alike). They will each be on their own schedule and that is completely okay.

Two Months
- Begins to smile at people
- Tries to look at parent
- Coos, makes gurgling sounds
- Turns head toward sounds
- Begins to follow things with eyes and recognize people at a distance
- Can hold head up and begins to push up when lying on tummy
- Makes smoother movements with arms and legs

Inform your doctor if your child:
- Doesn't respond to loud sounds
- Doesn't watch things as they move

*Source—Centers for Disease Control and Prevention

- Doesn't smile at people
- Doesn't bring hands to mouth
- Can't hold head up when pushing up while on tummy

Four Months

- Smiles spontaneously, especially at people
- Copies some movements and facial expressions, like smiling or frowning
- Begins to babble
- Babbles with expression and copies sounds he hears
- Reaches for toy with one hand
- Uses hands and eyes together, such as seeing a toy and reaching for it
- Follows moving things with eyes from side to side
- Holds head steady, unsupported
- Pushes down on legs when feet are on a hard surface
- Can hold a toy and shake it and swing at dangling toys
- Brings hands to mouth
- When lying on stomach, pushes up to elbows

Inform your doctor if your child:

- Doesn't watch things as they move
- Doesn't smile at people
- Can't hold her head steady
- Has trouble moving one or both eyes in all directions
- Doesn't push down with legs when feet are placed on a hard surface

Six Months

- Knows familiar faces and begins to know if someone is a stranger
- Likes to play with others, especially parents
- Responds to other people's emotions and often seems happy
- Responds to sounds by making sounds
- Strings vowels together when babbling ("ah," "eh," "oh") and likes taking turns with parent while making sounds

- Responds to own name
- Looks around at things nearby
- Brings things to mouth
- Shows curiosity about things and tries to get things that are out of reach
- Begins to pass things from one hand to the other
- Rolls over in both directions (front to back, back to front)
- Begins to sit without support
- When standing, supports weight on legs and might bounce
- Rocks back and forth, sometimes crawling backward before moving forward

Inform your doctor if your child:
- Shows no affection for caregivers
- Doesn't try to get things that are in reach
- Doesn't respond to sounds around him
- Has difficulty getting things to his mouth
- Doesn't make vowel sounds ("ah," "eh," "oh")
- Doesn't roll over in either direction
- Doesn't laugh or make squealing sound
- Seems very stiff, but tight muscles
- Seems very floppy, like a rag doll

Nine Months
- May be afraid of strangers
- May be clingy with familiar adults
- Has favorite toys
- Understands "no"
- Makes a lot of different sounds like "mamamama" and "babababa"
- Copies sounds and gestures of others
- Uses fingers to point at things
- Watches the path of something as it falls
- Looks for things he sees you hide

- Plays peekaboo
- Puts things in her mouth
- Moves things smoothly from one hand to the other
- Picks up things like Cheerios between thumb and index finger
- Stands, holding on
- Can get into sitting position
- Sits without support
- Pulls to stand
- Crawls

Inform your doctor if your child:
- Doesn't bear weight on legs
- Doesn't sit with help
- Doesn't babble ("mama," "baba," "dada")
- Doesn't play any games involving back-and-forth play
- Doesn't respond to name
- Doesn't seem to recognize familiar people
- Doesn't look where you point
- Doesn't transfer toys from one hand to another

One Year
- Is shy or nervous with strangers
- Cries when Mom or Dad leaves
- Has favorite things and people
- Shows fear in some situations
- Hands you a book when he wants to hear a story
- Repeats sounds or actions to get attention
- Puts out arm or leg to help with dressing
- Plays games such as peekaboo and pat-a-cake
- Responds to simple spoken requests
- Uses simple gestures, like shaking head "no" or waving "bye-bye"
- Makes sounds with changes in tone (sounds more like speech)
- Says "mama" and "dada" and exclamations like "uh-oh!"

- Tries to say words you say
- Explores things in different ways, like shaking, banging, throwing
- Finds hidden things easily
- Looks at the right picture or thing when it's named
- Copies gestures
- Starts to use things correctly; for example, drinks from a cup, brushes hair
- Bangs two things together
- Puts things in a container, takes things out of a container
- Lets things go without help
- Pokes with index (pointer) finger
- Follows simple directions like "pick up the toy"
- Gets to a sitting position without help
- Pulls up to stand, walks holding on to furniture ("cruising")
- May take a few steps without holding on
- May stand alone

Inform your doctor if your child:
- Doesn't crawl
- Can't stand when supported
- Doesn't search for things you hide
- Doesn't point at things
- Doesn't learn gestures like waiting or shaking head
- Loses skills they once had
- Doesn't say single words like "mama or "dada"

CHAPTER 8

feed me

O NE OF THE TOPICS THAT EXPECTANT PARENTS OF TWINS WORRY about the most is how they will feed their babies. First, there is the hot-button topic of the breast vs. bottle, and twin mamas often stress about whether or not they'll be able to find the time, patience, and milk supply to nurse. While this is a legitimate concern, I want all mothers of twins to know that if it is important to you, it is possible in most cases to nurse twins for as long as you like. That said, if the idea of nursing two babies makes you want to tear your hair out or there is another legitimate reason for you not to nurse, I will be the first person to tell you that it's okay. You have to do what is best for you and trust that whatever is best for you will ultimately be best for your babies.

Once you've decided whether to breast- or bottle-feed your twins, you must figure out the logistics of feeding the two of them at once. This is something that parents of twins are alone in experiencing, and it may seem completely overwhelming to you now. But you should cherish this precious time to feed and nurture your two babies! While it may feel clumsy at first, with the tips in this chapter, you'll soon feel so comfortable feeding both babies that you'll wonder why the idea ever made you so nervous. No, really. Let's dig in.

Solo or Tandem

You may have known all of your life that when you had kids of your own one day, you would do everything you could to breast-feed them. On the other hand, you may be the type of mother who never intended to nurse and who always felt completely comfortable with the idea of feeding her baby formula. Either way, finding out that you are having twins has probably changed your image of how you will feed your offspring more than a little bit. This is something that secretly saddens many mothers of twins. They see their singleton counterparts picking up their one baby in a park and easily putting her to the breast to begin a peaceful, euphoric nursing session. Birds chirp, the sun shines, and mother and baby are united in a beautiful bonding moment.

No such moment exists for mothers of twins. Even if you choose to nurse and want to try nursing one baby at a time, there will always be another hungry baby waiting for his or her turn. But although you can't have the exact experience that you might have imagined, you can have an equally beautiful time feeding your babies. You just have to let go of the image you had of blissfully feeding your one baby. Say good-bye to it, and then we can move on to the reality of feeding twins.

It's just not realistic to exclusively nurse or bottle-feed *one baby at a time* unless you are bottle-feeding only and can count on extra help at every feeding. If you feed them one at a time, there will always be another hungry baby sitting there, waiting for his or her turn. When they are newborns, babies need to eat approximately twelve times a day. That's twenty-four feedings if done separately! If you allot twenty minutes per feeding (a low estimate), you'll be feeding a baby for eight hours a day. I certainly hope you're convinced that tandem is where it's at. This chapter will give you tips on how to do it successfully.

Breast or Formula (or Both)

I won't ever try to convince a mother to breast-feed if she doesn't want to. A lot of moms feel pressured to nurse, and the health benefits for mothers and their babies have already been well documented. I think it's really great if you can nurse your twins, but if you can't, it's okay. Formula may be second-best, but it is a very good second-best option and one that is completely fine for your baby. If breast-feeding doesn't work out for you for whatever reason, don't feel guilty. You should not breast-feed if it's at the expense of your own health or sanity.

Sometimes moms need to give each other permission to do what's best for them. I am definitely not "anti-breast-feeding," but I am strongly "pro mom." It is much more important that you stay healthy and sane in order to raise your children than it is to breast-feed. I may get a lot of flack for saying that, but it's true. And that's really how I feel. I believe that my need to breast-feed my children contributed to my postpartum depression. If somebody had just given me permission and said, "Nat, you need to take care of yourself and then the twins," I think my early parenting experience would've been much better.

The most important thing is that you are healthy and happy so that you can care for your munchkins. If you are losing your mind because you are so stressed out about nursing, then you might be better off bottle-feeding. On the other hand, if you give up on nursing too soon and go on to regret it and feel guilty about it for years down the line, then you probably should have tried harder to keep nursing. Unless you are completely dead set against nursing or have a medical reason not to nurse, you should give it a solid try, so it's always an option. Breast milk operates on a supply-and-demand system. If there is no demand, your milk will dry up. So if there is even the slightest possibility you'd like to breast-feed, you should try to nurse, or at least pump if having them latch on isn't working out, as soon as the babies are born.

If you want to breast-feed, or are open to the idea of it, set small goals for yourself. Never say, "I'm going to nurse the twins for their first year." You'll only be setting yourself up for failure and heartache if something happens and you can no longer continue to nurse. The truth is that you won't know exactly how you'll feel about breast-feeding until after your babies are born. You may hate the idea now but be overcome by an instinctual urge to put those babies to your breast the first time you hold them. You never know. My best advice is to keep an open mind and learn all you can about both ways of feeding your babies now so that you have options later.

Don't forget that many mothers successfully feed their children with a combination of breast milk and formula, which may be a "best of both worlds" scenario. Some mothers simply don't produce enough milk to exclusively breast-feed two. Any milk you can produce is great. If it's just a small amount, you might want to consider breast-feeding one baby per feeding and giving a formula-filled bottle to the other and then switch. But know that it isn't unusual to need to supplement with a little formula to feed your babies all they need for the day. Despite what some extremists may lead you to believe, feeding your children does not have to be an all-or-nothing proposition. You have many choices and all of them will serve your children just fine. In the first months, your only job is to take care of yourself and do what feels right to you so that you can mother them the best that you can.

Tandem Nursing Your Twins

Welcome to the wild world of nursing two babies! Nursing is natural and will eventually feel relaxing, but in the beginning, it's work. In fact, the job starts before your twins are even born, because you should buy some lanolin cream to have on hand for your nipples. I recommend Lansinoh cream—it is a natural balm that protects your nipples from your babies' latch or a pump's grip that will wreak havoc on your nipples if you're not prepared.

Nursing in the Hospital

Once the twins are born, you will want to get them on the breast as soon as possible. At this point, your milk will not have come in yet. Instead, you will be producing a thicker, yellowish product called colostrum. (You may notice this colostrum leaking from your nipples toward the end of your pregnancy, which is normal.) Colostrum is a liquid that will secrete from your nipples in the same fashion as breast milk. Colostrum is different from breast milk in a few ways:

- It's more yellow in color.
- It's lower in fat.
- It's higher in protein.
- It's rich with antibodies to protect your newborns.

You will produce less colostrum than milk and you will only produce this in the very beginning of your new-mom experience. You only need to produce a tiny bit since your baby's stomach is so small at birth that it can barely hold an ounce of liquid. The small amount of colostrum that you'll produce will be enough to satisfy your twins until your milk comes in (usually around the third to fifth day postpartum).

If you pump after the birth instead of breast-feeding, don't be surprised by the tiny amount of colostrum that you get. It may be only a pea-sized amount. Make sure that the twins get that fed to them by a bottle, with a dripper, or even off your finger. I've seen parents throw out the colostrum, thinking that it's not enough to be worthwhile, which just kills me. Your spouse should bring the babies the colostrum if you are in recovery and feed it to the twins off his finger. (Try to give them equal amounts!)

Continue to nurse your babies on demand while you're in the hospital, as this is what will cause your milk to come in. When it does—watch out! You will probably be painfully engorged for about forty-eight hours, but continue to nurse through this and trust that it will settle down as your milk supply is established. If you cannot nurse during this time, just pump every couple of hours to establish your supply. You can feed your babies formula in the meantime, which may be necessary if they are in the NICU, born premature, or if your doctors feel it's best. As long as you continue to stimulate your breasts via either a pump or the babies themselves, your milk should come in by the third to fifth day.

Some hospitals have policies about the babies getting formula if your milk hasn't come in within twenty-four or forty-eight hours, but breast-feeding advocates would never recommend this. Again, listen to your doctor and make an informed decision. A lot of this will depend on what happened during the birth and whether or not the twins were born premature.

Remember to practice, practice, practice nursing while you are in the hospital! At first, you *do* want to practice nursing each baby separately, so that you can feel confident. But definitely try tandem nursing in the hospital if you can. Have the nurses and the lactation consultant watch you nurse so that they can point out any latch problems or physical abnormalities that may have to be addressed. Once you head home, you'll basically be on your own, so take advantage of having access to these professionals now.

Nursing at Home

Once you are at home with your twins, you can really settle in and get down to the business of nursing your babies. And it will surely feel like serious business at first, but remember that it does get easier with time. When it's time to feed some babies, the very first thing you have to do is get prepared.

Set your breast-feeding area with the supplies you need during feeding time. Everything should be within arm's reach when you are feeding your duo. Typical supplies are:

- a glass of water (or water bottle)
- telephone
- TV remote
- something to read
- light snack

Having these items on hand will ensure that you will not have to stop in the middle of a feeding to get anything. Also, you should go to the bathroom yourself before you begin the entire process.

After you are ready to start your feeding I personally suggest that you swaddle your babies during the first few weeks. When bottle-feeding, it doesn't seem to make much of a difference, but I humbly believe that swaddled babies nurse better. Check out my tips for swaddling on pages 137–139.

Once one baby is changed and swaddled, bring him or her into the room where you're planning to nurse and put her down somewhere safe while you go back and change and swaddle her twin. Place both of them safely next to you and strap on your breast-feeding pillow. You will want to nurse somewhere big and comfortable, such as your bed, the couch, or the floor. Unfortunately, you won't usually fit on a rocking chair or glider with two babies and that giant breast-feeding pillow, so let's say you'll be nursing on the couch. You're going to get the baby who is the better latcher to latch on first. Don't worry—once you start nursing, you will know right away which baby is the better latcher.

Breast-feeding Positions

Try each of these positions several times before deciding which ones work best for you. One might not work at first but may later become your favorite. Remember that different positions work at different stages of your twins' lives. There are also plenty of variations of any and all of these positions, and so I strongly encourage you to keep experimenting to find the one that fits you and your twins best. Remember that when you use pillows for positioning during breast-feeding, you must carefully watch your twins. If at any time you are concerned that their breathing might be in danger or if they look distressed, be sure to change positions to protect their safety and well-being.

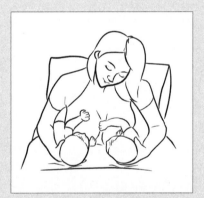

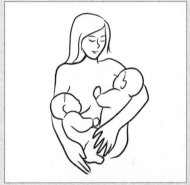

Double Clutch or Double "Football" Hold. *Each baby is facing you while they are latched on. Their bodies are tucked under your arms and your hands are supporting their heads. With a double breast-feeding pillow, this is the most popular feeding position for newborn twins.*

Double Cradle Hold. *Holding both babies as you would if they were individually cradled in your arms, allow them to latch on and simply overlap their bodies. If they are swaddled this will be simpler since you can avoid one kicking the other by accident. This position provides an opportunity for the twins to interact with each other during a feeding in a way that the Double Clutch does not.*

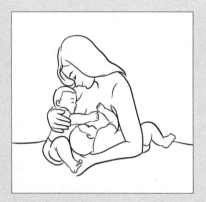

Cradle Clutch Position. *This position is the best of both worlds—it combines the Cradle Hold with the Clutch Hold.*

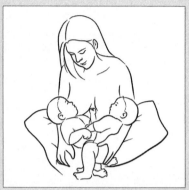

Criss Cross. *This hold is used by positioning your twins in an "x" fashion against your body with one in front of the other. This might be best done in bed, or on the couch with plenty of support both for the mother and babies.*

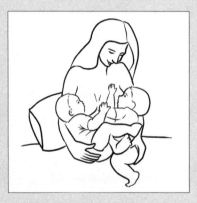

Reclining Criss Cross. *This position might be best in an almost full recline position. With a minimal amount of propping to elevate your head, and plenty of pillows on each side of your body, you might find that this position is most comfortable in the middle of the night (if someone can bring you two diaper-changed babies). This position will allow each child to almost lie on top of you while feeding.*

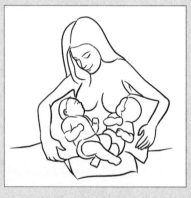

Cradle Cross Position. *This position combines the Cross Position with the popular Cradle Hold. While it might be a bit challenging at first, practice makes perfect for this and all the breast-feeding positions.*

> *From the MOM Squad:* "Give it a chance. If you can get through the first two weeks, you are probably completely set and will have few, if any, problems thereafter. If it's not for you, don't feel guilty. You need to do what's best for you and your family, and guilt is never the best for you and them." —Katie M.

Once that baby is latched on in the football hold, tuck a rolled-up receiving blanket underneath her for additional support. Now she's not going anywhere and you can focus on getting her twin to latch. Give him a pep talk, do whatever you have to do, and then get him on the other breast in the same position. Place a rolled-up blanket underneath him, too. Now they are both secure and you are completely hands-free! You can eat a sandwich, read the newspaper, or play on your iPad. (Stay away from hot soup or coffee, though, and try not to get crumbs in the twins' eyes.)

One important thing to remember about nursing twins is that one baby will almost definitely be a better latcher and also a better drinker. Because of the supply-and-demand system, if you always put the better drinker on the same breast, that breast will grow larger than the other one due to greater demand for milk. The way to resolve this is to *alternate* breasts at each feeding. Unlike with singletons, you will only feed each *baby on one breast per feeding*, and then switch sides for the next feeding. Don't trust yourself to remember this! Just get a simple bracelet or a hair tie and keep it on the wrist where Baby B (Think B = Bracelet) ate last. They also sell fancy bra pins for this purpose, but it's not really necessary to buy those.

And that's it! Sounds simple, right? Well, it can be, and if you stick with it, eventually it will be.

Potential Nursing Pitfalls

Here are a few common nursing problems and how you can prevent and heal from them.

Milk Not "Coming In"

The signal for the breasts to make milk has to do with the placenta leaving the uterus. Moms who have Cesarean deliveries often have to wait longer for their milk to come in. After a vaginal delivery, it is common to see the milk come in on day two or three. With a C-section, it is more common to see it come in on day four or five. In some cases, it can take a week. Frequent nursing or stimulation with a hospital-grade breast pump may help bring the milk in faster. Also, mothers who have had babies before may produce milk faster. When a mother is not making milk, it is usually because she is not stimulating enough or at all. It is *very rare* for a mother not to make milk, but if you feel that this may be the case for you, speak with your doctor.

Low Supply

If you're concerned about your milk supply, call a lactation consultant or nurse-practitioner. There are herbal supplements like fenugreek and Mother's Milk Tea that you can take to boost your supply, but you should get your doctor's okay first. Some people say that drinking a pint of Guinness every day helps boost their supply—it's up to you if you want to try it. Remember above all else that breast-feeding is supply and demand, so if you aren't producing enough, the easiest remedy is to nurse or pump more.

Skin-to-skin contact is also very good for helping you produce milk, so take off your shirt and snuggle with your naked babies. Your instincts will likely kick in and you'll start to feel a little tingle in your boobs. Your supply may dip when the babies go through a growth spurt since they often demand to feed more often—every two hours instead of every three. Follow the babies' lead, and in a few days your supply will increase. And be sure to eat and drink enough!

Mastitis

This happens with singletons, too, but not as often as when breast-feeding twins. Mastitis is a breast infection that occurs when a milk duct in your breast becomes blocked. It is harmless for the babies, but it makes the mother feel as sick as if she had the flu. You'll need antibiotics if it's bad enough, so call your doctor if you come down with a fever ASAP. You can prevent mastitis if you catch the blocked duct early on, so be on the lookout for any hard, painful lumps on your breasts and call your doctor right away if you find one.

Painful Nipples

I'm very sorry to tell you this, but they may crack and they may bleed. Remember to put that lanolin cream on every chance you get, and stock up on nursing pads so that it doesn't get all over your clothes. Another trick is to soak your nipples in salt water three times a day. This sounds crazy, I know, but it really speeds up healing. Sore, cracked nipples can be very painful, but once you've ruled out any latching issues, just keep going and the nursing will get easier and more comfortable over time.

Engorgement

Delivering my twins was weird, but having milk shoot out of my breasts onto the walls of the shower was much weirder. There are many reasons that you might get engorged—when the milk first comes in and your supply is being established, or if you're dealing with a plugged duct or mastitis. When you're engorged, your breasts will become hard and painful. The best way to relieve this is to get some milk out. Pump a little or hand express (by just pressing down on your breasts), but be careful about pumping too much, because you'll only be stimulating your breasts to produce more. The best way to find relief is to stand in the warm shower and let the milk leak out, as this is soothing and nonstimulating. But it is weird at first. You'll get used to it.

> ***From the MOM Squad:*** *"Keep with it. One tip that saved my life was that one of my twins wouldn't latch because milk wasn't available right away (we'd struggled for ten weeks). I was told to nurse in the shower. The water dripping down my breast kept the baby interested until the milk let down and our prayers were answered!" —Amber D.*

Your Breast-feeding Diet

Although you have to be sure to eat well while you're pregnant with twins, you have to eat almost twice as consciously when you're breast-feeding. You must hydrate and eat enough food to stay nourished so you can produce milk for two babies. That is a lot. Creating breast milk burns calories, in the neighborhood of 20 calories an ounce. That means that if you're nursing twins you need to consume an additional 1,000 calories a day. This is your job now.

Also remember that the babies eat what you eat. This doesn't mean that you have to drastically restrict your diet, but you should be mindful of what you're putting into your body. Watch out for your babies' reaction to what you eat. If you have a spicy curry and then they act fussy the entire next day, they probably didn't dig the curry. When it's time for them to start solids, your babies will actually recognize and prefer the spices that you ate when you were nursing them, so it's a good idea to eat a varied diet to try and avoid having obnoxiously picky toddlers. (I said try.) If you're an adventurous eater, it's more likely that they will be adventurous eaters.

When it comes to caffeine and alcohol, it's all about moderation. One or two cups of coffee a day is fine (and, in all honesty, necessary). As for alcohol, I do not recommend that you get wasted, but if you do, there are three things that you can do.

(1) First, you can pump and dump, which means that you pump at the next feed and then toss all the milk out, just to be safe. (2) There are strips you can buy that you can dunk in your breast milk to test the alcohol content (seriously). Even if you have a drink or two, the babies will not be affected unless your blood alcohol content is elevated. (3) If you are out and you don't have a pump on you, you can manually pump to ward off engorgement. When you get engorged, it's Mother Nature telling you that it's time to go home and feed your babies, so put the drink down, throw in the towel, and go home. But don't feel guilty. Sometimes a night out with the girls can go a long way in helping you be a better mom!

Pumping

Even if you plan to stay home full-time and exclusively nurse your twins, chances are that at some point, you're going to want (or need) to pump. Pumping is important (though not always necessary) for establishing milk supply in the beginning, and later on it is essential if you ever want to take a break and have someone else feed the babies so that you can leave their sides for a few hours and get your hair done. (Spoiler alert—you will.)

When you're pumping for twins, I highly suggest that you get a double electric pump or rent a hospital-grade pump. Some singleton moms can get away with a single battery-operated pump or even a hand pump, but I wouldn't try it. Remember to check with your insurance company to see if this expense is covered (see chapter 1 for more details on this).

If you want to pump in order to start building a supply of breast milk for your twins, you need to create a pumping schedule based on when they eat. If you start pumping at random times throughout the day, you risk eating into the twins' next feeding (pun intended). Start by pumping for ten minutes after each feeding. Every time the twins eat, put them down afterward, pump for ten minutes, and that's it. Even if you don't get much milk out, don't be tempted to pump more than this or you'll leach from your own supply. Just keep a bottle in the fridge and keep pumping into that bottle over the course of a day. Even if you only get two ounces each time you pump, you'll have at least a full feeding at the end of the day, and if

---

TWINIVERSITY TIP: A PUMPING SCHEDULE

When do you pump? If you are not making enough milk on your own, pumping is a much more efficient way to get your breasts to produce the maximum amount of milk. A pump is never tired, always extracts milk at the level you set it for, and is never cranky. Also, you might want to pump so you can leave behind milk for the twins if you're returning to work or planning to be away from them for an extended period of time.

you keep up this schedule, you'll begin producing and pumping more and more because of the additional demand.

When you do leave a bottle of pumped milk behind, it is important that you "make up for it" by pumping while you're away from the twins. Not only will this be good for maintaining your supply, but you will probably become engorged if you skip feedings. The same thing goes for when you return to work. Because it's supply and demand, you need to pump when the babies should be eating if you want to keep up your supply. It should take about twenty minutes each time you pump, so it is a big commitment. There are now laws about providing a comfortable place for you to pump at work, so look into that, or you can just pump in your office if you have a door. You can pump and work if you purchase one of those special pumping bras (or just buy a cheap tank top with a shelf bra and cut two holes in the shelf portion of it) to support the pump so you can be hands-free to get tasks done.

Here are some quick numbers regarding pumped breast milk and how long it stays fresh:

- In the fridge—five days
- In the freezer—six months to a year (depending on your freezer)
- On the counter (or in your bag)—five hours
- Once it's defrosted—twenty-four hours

TWINIVERSITY TIP

Some moms (like myself) opted to exclusively pump their breast milk and bottle-feed their twins the pumped milk. This is a growing trend within the multiple birth community since this option gives you the flexibility to have others help feed the twins while providing your own milk for their nourishment.

Top Ten Tips from the Pro

For more breast-feeding tips and troubleshooting, I asked Sheri Bayles, RN, BSN, LCCE, IBCLC, for her top ten tips for successful twin nursing.

1. On day of delivery, make sure to nurse and/or stimulate your breasts with a hospital-grade breast pump for the first forty-eight hours every three hours <u>no fail</u>. This lets your body know that you want to make milk quickly. It also ensures a good milk supply in the future.

2. Keep a feeding journal every day to keep track of what is going in and coming out of the babies (see Appendix B).

3. Tandem nursing (feeding both at the same time) is time efficient, but I only recommend trying it when you feel confident and comfortable nursing each baby individually.

4. Feed your babies on a schedule every two to three hours (from start to start) around the clock. It makes life more manageable and predictable.

5. Once the babies reach 6 pounds (unless otherwise recommended by your pediatrician), the babies may call the schedule from midnight to 6 a.m. If one baby wakes up, wake the other to keep the feeds together.

6. If you want to stockpile some milk in the freezer for future breast milk bottles, pump both breasts immediately following your first three to four feeds in the morning. I recommend you start doing this the day you come home from the hospital.

7. Try to exclusively breast-feed the first two weeks without supplement or bottle-feeding. However, there are many exceptions to this recommendation—one being premature babies (see below).

8. Introducing bottles after two to four weeks allows the partner to get involved with the feedings and gives moms a break.

9. Mothers who breast-feed exclusively need to consume 3,500 to 4,000 calories a day to keep up with the demands of two babies. Don't worry. You are burning tons of calories, so the postpartum weight will come off.

10. Surround yourself with very supportive breast-feeding friends and family members.

Weaning Your Twins

When to wean your twins can be a difficult decision for many moms. I'm actually not sure if weaning is harder on the mom or the twins! The weaning process can happen at any time from a few weeks after the babies are born to years later. The process itself can take days, weeks, or months. It all depends on you and your family. There is no one perfect way to do this, but there are ways to make it easier on you and the babies when the time comes. Here are my best tips for making weaning as painless a transition as possible for all of you.

Go Gradual

Start by dropping one feeding every few days. When you drop each feeding, replace the breast milk with a glass of milk (or formula if they are under a year) and a snack and replace the time that you normally would've spent nursing with snuggling or story time. This way, the twins won't feel like they're losing out on their quality time with you. Going "cold turkey" would probably be a very difficult transition for your twins and make them feel disconnected from you and each other. Slow and steady wins the race during the weaning process. I also suggest dropping the last feeding of the day *last*, as the bedtime feeding provides a great deal of comfort as well as nutrition.

Put Your Twins in the Driver's Seat

If you're not in a rush to wean, you can try letting the twins decide when they're ready to wean instead of making the decision for them. The downside of this technique could be that the twins never make this tough decision, or one decides to continue breast-feeding while the other one stops. If this happens, the one who's no longer nursing might start to feel jealous of the time that you're spending with the one who still is. Just be careful and make sure that you spend one-on-one time with each of them to make up for this.

Talk It Out

Depending on how old your twins are when you wean, they might understand if you tell them that your milk needs to go "bye-bye." Some young babies are mature enough to understand this, so it's worth a shot to talk it through with them.

Get Dad Involved

This is the perfect time to get Dad more involved in feedings. During the times when you would normally nurse your twins, have your spouse offer them a bottle or cup of milk or just some cuddle time. It's not unusual for spouses to feel a disconnect with their children when their wives are breast-feeding since babies spend so much of their time eating. Use weaning as a good excuse to bring Dad closer to his twins.

Experiment with Bottles and Cups

If you're weaning before your babies are able to hold a cup and you're having difficulties with getting them to drink from a bottle, you may want to experiment with different types of bottles and nipples. Some babies prefer silicone nipples while others like latex. Try a few and let your babies decide which ones they like best. Straw cups or sippy cups might work, too.

Manage Your Emotions

The weaning process can be very emotional for some mothers. It's a major time of transition from one stage to another in your children's lives, and it can take a toll on you. Try to make the most of your freedom from nursing by planning some special time for yourself while your husband feeds the babies.

> **From the MOM Squad:** *"Don't stress about nursing because it doesn't work for everyone. Yes, it is great if you can, but formula works well, too. I wound up doing both and it really took a lot of pressure off me."* —*Erica D.*

Avoid Engorgement

Most moms will experience some engorgement while weaning. If you need to express some breast milk with a pump or even your hands, do what you have to do to make sure that you stay comfortable. Just pump enough milk to be comfortable, but not enough to mimic a whole feeding.

If you're having a lot of difficulty with engorgement, cabbage leaves can be your best friend. Apparently, there is an acid in green cabbage leaves that produces an anti-irritant that helps dilate your capillaries, making it easier for milk to flow and allowing you to get just enough milk out to be comfortable without the assistance of the babies.

Note: If you have an allergy to cabbage or sulfur, do not use this method. Otherwise, simply take some green cabbage leaves (they must be green), crush them with your hands to release the enzymes, and place them inside your bra. Leave them there for twenty to thirty minutes, then remove and make a salad. I recommend a nice balsamic vinaigrette. Just kidding, of course; throw the used cabbage leaves in the trash. You can do this a few times a day to relieve your discomfort, but discontinue this process immediately if you experience any irritation.

Bottle-feeding Your Twins

The benefits of bottle-feeding your twins are pretty obvious—anyone can feed them at any time, there is a lot less guesswork because you know exactly how much each twin is eating each time they eat, and it is physically a lot less demanding for you. The cons are just as obvious—there is a lot more time spent messing around with bottles, more stuff to clean, more to bring with you when you dare to leave the house with the twins, and some babies have bad reactions to certain formulas, which can be extra annoying since your twins could end up taking two different formulas. But if you decide that your twins will be fed with formula (or if Mother Nature decides for you), there are ways to make it as simple and painless as anything involved in parenting twins.

The first thing to know is that powdered formula is just as good as the liquid kind. A lot of parents assume that the liquid formulas are better because that's what they use at the hospital, but the liquid formulas are much more expensive and the powder really is nutritionally the same. Powdered formulas are also much more convenient than liquid. When you wake up in the morning, or even the night before, fill up the day's bottles with just the powder for each feeding. Then boil a pot of water and put it in a pitcher, and then anytime you need a bottle during the day, you have a sterilized pitcher of water to fill up the bottles with. You don't have to warm it up or anything; room temperature is fine. Just shake it up and you're all set and ready to feed some babies.

Remember to make your bottles exactly according to the instructions. Don't add a bonus scoop to make it thicker or to attempt to get the babies to sleep longer.

When it comes to nipples, the babies will be using Level 1 nipples when they come home from the hospital. A lot of parents forget to upgrade to Level 2 at the appropriate time. One clue is if it starts taking the babies longer than twenty minutes to complete a feeding. This means that they're not really hungry or else the nipple is too small and they're having trouble getting the formula out. What bottles should you use? Every baby has his or her preference, but my kids hugely preferred Dr. Brown's in the beginning, and these bottles helped immensely with my daughter's reflux.

Two Babies, Two Formulas

If one baby has reflux, an allergy, or another medical issue, he or she may need a special formula. The best trick for keeping the two different formulas apart is to put a little nail polish on the bottom of the bottle with the special formula. This won't come off in the dishwasher and is a great little cheat. Another twin parent's godsend is Mabel's Labels, which are great for labeling anything for your kids but especially bottles because they are also dishwasher safe. You can also buy special bands that go around the bottle to help you tell them apart.

If one or both of your children have to be fed with special predigested formulas, be warned that they can be extremely expensive, but it is likely that your insurance will cover them as if they were medicine. This is something that nobody else will tell you! The predigested formulas can cost you sixteen dollars a day without insurance or just your copayment for the entire month with insurance. No, that does not mean that your other twin should be on the same formula just because it's covered, but it does mean that you shouldn't stock up on formula too soon. You never know what's going to happen. To find out if your formula is covered, ask your pediatrician or call your insurance company.

Tandem Bottle-feeding

Bottle-feeding twins is a bit more straightforward than breast-feeding, but you still want to have all your supplies ready ahead of time. These will include your bottles (obviously), two rolled-up receiving blankets, and your bouncy seats. Most twin moms find the bouncy seats to be the best place to tandem bottle-feed twins. You can also use car seats and eventually move on to Bumbo seats or high chairs, but bouncy seats are cheap, stackable, and work perfectly. The receiving blankets work as a head support when the babies are little and their heads are still wobbly. You can buy a fancy head-support cushion, too, but a cheapo blanket works just fine. Just roll it up like a giant cigar, make an upside-down U, and rest their head on the inner portion of that U. Make sure it is secure and can't cover the baby's face. As a bonus, receiving blankets are superabsorbent and will catch any drool or spit-up that happens while the babies are eating.

Next, you simply sit on the floor facing the babies in their bouncy seats with a bottle in each hand and feed the twins. No, this isn't as cuddly as breast-feeding, but you can still turn it into quality time by singing or talking to the babies as they eat. My husband would play loud music while he fed our twins and they all had a blast. Find a way to make it special for you.

You may find that one twin has to burp while the other one is still eating. In this case, just do your best to keep feeding the one baby while burping the other. No matter what, please do not use a bottle prop. Bottle props basically prop the bottle up on the baby's chest so that you don't need to hold it for him. This is a controversial topic, but I am very opposed to bottle props, because the baby can choke if too much liquid flows into his mouth, and he cannot remove it himself.

Starting Solids

When your twins are four to six months old, your pediatrician will probably give you the okay to start feeding your babies solid food. At this stage, the word "solid" isn't really accurate. Your twins' first foods should be quite liquidy. Starting to eat solids is really more about learning to eat food off a spoon instead of out of a nipple. This is a really fun and messy milestone for you and your babies, so get plenty of bibs ready, charge up the camera, and get yourself psyched to have fun making a mess!

Moms always ask me what the best first food is to feed their twins. If your twins have any allergies or health concerns, rice cereal (made with either breast milk or formula) is the safest, most hypoallergenic food that you can feed them. However, it gets boring really fast and can be quite . . . binding. We moved to baby oatmeal that first week. It is more nutritionally sound than the "filler" that rice provides. Two other great choices for your first attempt at feeding your babies solids are bananas or avocado. Avocado isn't sold in a jar, but it's a fantastic first baby food. Both bananas and avocados can easily be made into baby food at home. Since your twins won't likely be eating much during their first forays into solids, you can make a small amount in a blender and thin the food out with breast milk or formula until it is wet enough to hardly resemble a solid at all. It's really more soupy than anything.

Once you get going with feeding your babies solids, you will realize how quickly you start going through those tiny glass jars of baby food! With two babies, the cost of baby food can add up really fast. This is one of the reasons that I highly recommend making your own baby food at home. Not only does it drastically reduce costs, but it gives you complete control over the foods and ingredients that you are feeding your twins.

Making baby food is not hard at all. It also doesn't have to be all or nothing. You can make some baby food yourself and then supplement with jars or pouches when you're out of the house. That said, some types of baby food are not very easy or cost-effective to make yourself. It can be tricky to get the right consistency out of green beans or meats, so it might make sense to use jars if you want to feed your babies these foods. Depending on where you live, it might be difficult to find fresh ingredients at different times of the year. These are good reasons to supplement with store-bought baby foods from time to time.

Two of the easiest and cost-effective foods to make at home are carrots and sweet potatoes. Just peel them, steam them until they are soft, and then puree, adding enough water to get the right consistency. Use the steaming liquid, which is full of vitamins from the veggies! Once you master these two, get creative and start blending up whatever fruits and vegetables you like to keep around the house. Remember when you are introducing solids to your twins to use the four-day rule anytime you feed them a new food. Wait four days after giving them a new food before trying another new food. This gives you a chance to look out for any possible allergic reactions. After four days with no reaction, feel free to introduce another new food.

Once your twins have tried a variety of new foods using the four-day wait rule and are eating well, you can start stocking up on their favorite foods by making big batches and freezing them. As the babies get older, you can start pureeing or finely chopping whatever you are making the rest of the family for dinner. This will be an easy way of transitioning them to table foods.

When we first introduced solids to our duo we started with "brunch." After their breakfast feeding we mixed a small bowl of oatmeal and formula/breast milk. From there, we introduced solids after most bottle-feedings. They had breakfast, lunch, and dinner after no time at all. We skipped rice cereal altogether since my daughter was having some constipation issues. This worked like a charm for us.

CHAPTER 9

schedule + sleep = sanity

CHEDULING AND SLEEP ARE TWO TOPICS THAT GO HAND IN HAND when it comes to your twins. You might assume that your babies will simply get tired and go to sleep at predictable times of the day and night, and that when you feed and bathe them doesn't have anything to do with how long or how well they will sleep. Let me set you straight right now. Putting your twins on a schedule is an important step toward your own sanity. The time before you do so will feel surreal and completely out of control.

If you don't believe me now, wait a few months. In fact, you'll have to wait a few months anyway, because you can't really put any baby on a sleep schedule until he or she's at least three or four months old. This time period can be painful and exhausting for singleton parents, but for parents of twins, it can be difficult to survive. Your two babies will be sleeping at random times of the day and night and often never at the same time for what will feel like forever. Yes, that means that you will be getting very little sleep, too. Hooray . . . sleep deprivation!

After those first few months, you'll realize that what you do (and don't do) and when you do it during the day has everything to do with how the twins sleep at night. Babies thrive on predictability, and it will become essential for you to take advantage of this by providing a reliable schedule by which they can set their internal clocks. This will also be the key for you to have some predictability to your days! So how do you get your twins on a schedule, and how will you ever get them to sleep through the night? This chapter will answer all of those questions, plus some you never would have thought to ask, by walking you through an ideal daily schedule for your twins and for you.

The First Few Weeks with Twins

The good news is, your newborns will sleep sixteen to eighteen hours per day, so you'll have a good chance to get acclimated to your new role as parent while they slumber. The bad news is, they usually only sleep in two- or three-hour chunks, and not always at the same time. To put it mildly, you might be a tiny bit tired. To put it plainly, you may be utterly exhausted unless you come up with a plan and recruit some help from family and friends, if possible. By the time they're a few months old, their sleeping patterns will become much more regular, but for a while, chaos will rule your household. Here is your survival guide for handling these first few crazy, precious, once-in-a-lifetime weeks.

Feeding

Since it's too early to put your twins on a sleep schedule, you can focus on creating a feeding schedule. Most full-term babies will be fine on a three-hour feeding schedule, whether they're breast- or bottle-fed. As tempting as it may be, I highly recommend that you don't let your babies sleep past this three-hour window. Newborns need to eat often, and these feedings also keep them hydrated. Plus, if they sleep through a feeding, they will make up for it later. (Ask your pediatrician when it's okay to start letting them sleep through feedings.) Also, this ensures that the twins will be eating at the same time, which will make your life much simpler! Wake them up when the clock is about to strike, change their diapers, and begin the feeding.

If you are exclusively breast-feeding, you may want to consider pumping a bit so your partner can take on one or two feedings. To do this, begin pumping twenty minutes before the feeding is scheduled to start, pump for twenty minutes, hand over some bottles to your spouse filled with your milk, and jump right back into bed. This may sound like a lot of work, but it's quicker than changing, feeding, burping, and resettling your babies. Plus, it gives your partner a chance to bond with the twins. If you don't want to pump before the feed, you can pump for ten minutes *after* each feed throughout the day and build up a supply to prevent having to get up at all, but wait until your supply is well established to start skipping feedings entirely. Remember that breast milk operates on a supply-and-demand schedule.

If you are bottle-feeding, prepare your bottles for the entire day ahead of time to save time. I recommend doing this throughout the twins' first several months. When it's time for a feeding, wake the twins, change their diapers, and give them bottles. To warm up a bottle, place it in a bowl of warm water. Don't ever use the microwave! It can heat up the core temperature of the formula (or breast milk) too much and burn your tiny tot, and also it kills some of the nutrients.

Some experts recommend feeding newborns "on demand" rather than on a schedule, but parents of twins often prefer to feed their twins on a schedule. Otherwise, feedings could literally take up your entire day. And having a routine can help make your day more predictable and therefore manageable. However, feeding on demand may very well work better for your family. Try both ways until you find what works best for you.

Playtime

After a feeding, your twins will be full and happy, so this is a good time to play with them. All babies need tummy time to help them develop their trunk muscles. Lay them flat on their tiny bellies, making sure their faces are to the side so they can breathe well. Try putting them right next to each other so they can see each other, and stay with them to make sure they are safe. Do this for five minutes at a time, several times a day.

Otherwise, your babies don't need much right now other than your love and affection. Hold them, smile and talk to them, sing to them, or even read them a story. (It's never too early.) There's nothing you have to do except enjoy them and they will enjoy you right back. When my twins were little I would set up a play mat, play Eye of the Tiger and place the babies on separate corners. I said, "In this corner we have Annaconda and over here we have Johnstrocity," and then faked a wrestling match (safely, of course). Enjoy this time when your kids can't roll their eyes at you!

Sleep Babies, Sleep

It's too early to sleep-train your twins (we'll get into this later in this chapter), but it's never too early to set up some good sleep habits. If you put your twins in their cribs drowsy but awake, they will get used to soothing themselves to sleep. If you see them yawn, rub their eyes, or even perform a "slow blink," hug and kiss them and put them down to sleep.

Here is what a day in the life might look like when your twins are brand-new (under three months). Please keep in mind that there really is no such thing as "normal" at this stage! This should only give you an idea of what could happen, not what necessarily will happen.

7 a.m.: Diaper change/feed
8 a.m.: Playtime/tummy time
8:30 a.m.: (if they stay awake) Nap
10 a.m.: Diaper change/feed
11 a.m.: Playtime/photo shoot

TWINIVERSITY TIP

Remember to always put your babies to sleep on their backs! This helps prevent SIDS (sudden infant death syndrome).

11:30 a.m.: Nap

1 p.m.: Diaper change/feed

2 p.m.: Go for a walk/nap in carriage

4 p.m.: Diaper change/feed

5 p.m.: Playtime

5:30 p.m.: Nap

7 p.m.: Diaper change/feed

7:45 pm.: Bath time/sponge bath

8:30 p.m.: Nap

10 p.m.: Diaper change/feed and right back to sleep

1 a.m.: Diaper change/feed and right back to sleep

4 a.m.: Diaper change/feed and right back to sleep

7 a.m.: Start a new day

To Sleep-Train, Perchance to Dream

Sleep training is a controversial topic among parents. In case you are unfamiliar with this term, sleep training essentially means teaching your children how to comfort themselves so that they can put themselves to sleep. Meaning that you do not rock, nurse, sing, or bounce your babies to sleep, but instead put them in their cribs awake and let them learn how to fall asleep themselves. Dr. Richard Ferber first popularized this concept, and so some people call it "Ferberizing" your babies. Another term for this method is, "cry it out," because, yes, there will be some crying involved.

But when you use these methods, you are not really training your babies to "sleep," but rather to soothe themselves. When babies are very little, they need help settling down to sleep, and you will instinctively find yourself rocking, singing, or nursing your babies to sleep. But it becomes much more difficult to settle your babies down the line at three and four months when they are heavier, alert, and more easily distracted.

Around this age, the more you need to intervene to get your babies to sleep, the more you will have to continue intervening, because every time the babies wake (or even become semiawake and start to babble or cry mildly) during the night, they will need you to come and help get them back to sleep. If they are able to fall asleep themselves, they will be able to go back to sleep easily during wake-ups and eventually sleep through the night. This is where sleep training comes in. By the time your twins are four months old (sometimes sooner, sometimes later if they were born early), they will be neurologically capable of putting themselves to sleep. That doesn't mean that they will agree to do it! Babies are smart, and they will have gotten used to all of your wonderful soothing techniques. They will protest being put down awake, and by protest I mean cry. In his book *Healthy Sleep Habits, Happy Twins,* Dr. Marc Weissbluth clearly outlines how to teach your baby to fall asleep using sleep training methods. I highly recommend you read it.

Many parents are against sleep training on principle. They believe that it is cruel to let their babies cry for any extended period of time, cannot bear to listen to it, and fear that it will cause their babies irreparable harm. I was one of these parents. In fact, I waited nearly nine months to sleep-train my twins. I don't know what I thought would happen; I was afraid that they would spontaneously combust or something. But after nine months without any quality sleep for anyone in my home, I couldn't take it anymore. My husband finally convinced me to let them cry it out and we never looked back, except to wholeheartedly regret not doing it at least four months sooner.

When you and the twins are ready for sleep training, simply begin putting them down drowsy, but awake, at their scheduled nap and bedtimes (according to the schedule on pages 185–186). They will cry. What you do next can vary slightly, depending on the method of sleep training that you prefer to follow. The "rapid extinction" method tells you to let them cry for however long it takes until they fall asleep. After just a few days and nights of this, they will generally go to sleep without any crying, but it can be tough for parents to stick to. Another method is by gradually letting them get used to being alone and involves your going in to soothe the babies

> *From the MOM Squad:* "We started sleep training at around six months. It was probably the hardest thing I've ever done, but I'll tell anyone who'll listen that it was worth it. I think we did it at the right time. Any later, and it would have probably been more difficult. I may do it a month or so earlier with the next child." —Holly B.

without picking them up, patting or hushing, every five or ten minutes. You must decide which method is best for you. Talk it over with your spouse, agree on a plan, and stick with it together. This is a very personal parenting decision and it is vital for everyone caring for the twins to be on the same page.

The truth is that parents of twins generally sleep-train their babies more often and sooner than their singleton peers. Perhaps it's just easier for a singleton parent to deal with soothing their baby to sleep several times a day or night, or to handle an unpredictable schedule as determined by one baby. Resettling two babies is infinitely more difficult than one. If you are against sleep training, no worries. I mean it sincerely. But you might want to keep reading, anyway, just in case your plans change down the road. Remember that it's never too late to do this. You might wait three years and then decide that you can't take it anymore and decide to sleep-train. That's fine. The rest of you ask your pediatrician when your twins will be ready to be sleep trained (usually by around 12 pounds and twelve weeks), and then get excited about finally getting some sleep.

A Day in the Life of Five-Month-Old Twins

Once you've gotten through those first months, your babies can start to settle into a more consistent routine. We're going to work our way through a typical day and talk about each routine, starting first thing in the morning. Whether everything went perfectly last night and the babies slept all the way through or it was a total nightmare, each morning is a fresh start and an opportunity to reset. (No matter what, always congratulate yourself on making it through another day!) Here is a guide to keep in mind for how to structure your day. **Note:** This schedule does not contain a middle-of-the-night feeding. Speak to your doctor before dropping *any* feeding just to be sure it's appropriate for your duo.

7 a.m.—Morning Feeding

You will wake up at 7 a.m., the birds will be chirping, and the babies will be hungry. The first thing that you will do is feed them. We already talked about how to go about this, so you will simply tandem-feed the twins, either from the breast or bottles. Don't forget to change their diapers first.

7:30 a.m.—Easy Entertainment

Now it's 7:30, give or take, and the babies are in the best moods that they'll be in all day. They slept all night (right?), so they are well rested, and they just ate. They are at their peak, so take advantage of this so that you can get some stuff done.

Set up an area of your house like it is a gym for babies with several different "stations." These baby entertainment stations should include a baby swing, a bouncy seat with a toy bar attached, a floor mat with some dangly toys, some board books on a flat surface, and maybe a little toy piano or some musical toys. Then put each baby at a station and rotate them every ten minutes. For example, for round one put one baby in the swing and the other on the play mat. Double-check that everything is safe. Then go into the kitchen and set the timer for ten minutes, and then unload the dishwasher. Then go back into the living room, and rotate one baby into the bouncy seat and station the other on the floor with books. Set the timer for another ten minutes and then check your e-mail.

I'm sure you can see where this is going. You can easily fill ninety minutes this way. That's only nine rotations. Don't be tempted to get on the floor and hold the babies all morning. There will be plenty of time for that later (trust me). Instead, make sure that you take this opportunity to get yourself organized for the day. Have a cup of coffee, brush your teeth, pay your bills, get your diaper bag ready for the day (more on that later), and get your bottles ready for the day if you're bottle-feeding. However, safety first. Always make sure the babies are safe and secure at all times.

9 a.m.—Morning Nap

Yes, your twins will already be ready for a nap, and I'm sure you will be, too. Make sure that their room is set up to be a good sleep environment, meaning that the room is very dark (think about investing in blackout shades or even tape some heavy-duty black garbage bags to the windows), and has some form of white noise. This can be a fancy white noise machine, a fan, or even a radio set to static. In the winter, consider using a humidifier unless your home is normally very humid. When you begin sleep training, you will begin with this nap. Make sure that everyone is on

TWINIVERSITY TIP

Everyone always asks me, "Nat, won't the babies disturb each other with all that crying?" and, amazingly, the answer is no. This is something that would be different for two singleton babies or even two siblings close in age, but twins don't seem to wake each other with their crying. I'm not the baby whisperer and I don't speak Baby, but I know that in seven years, my twins have never woken each other up, even when they were screaming bloody murder. If you find that you aren't so lucky, and you want to try separating them and you have the room, then be our guest. The majority of Twiniversity parents find that there is no need to separate them, but you will need to separate yourself from them, especially if you're nursing. If you put me in a room filled with cheesesteaks, I certainly wouldn't be able to sleep, and if you're nursing, you smell that good to your babies. They will be able to smell you from across the room, so make sure that you are on the other side of the house when you are trying to get them to sleep, if possible.

board, and that means you, your spouse, your nanny, and any neighbors who are within earshot. If you live in an apartment building or share a two-family home, maybe even think about leaving your neighbors a pound of coffee beans and some earplugs with a note that says, "We are sleep training. Sorry for the noise. Love, The Twins." It won't hurt to have them on your side.

Before putting the twins down for the nap, make sure they are clean and the ideal sleep conditions are in place.

Once the stage is set, you will kiss their cheeks, swaddle them if necessary, put the babies in their crib, turn off the lights, and close the door. They might cry. That is okay. I have never known a child to injure him or herself from crying.

11 a.m.—Midmorning Feeding

No matter how long they cry, the twins will eventually go to sleep. Whether they actually slept for five minutes or two hours, you will need to get them up at 11 a.m. Eventually, they will probably sleep for those entire two hours (or close to it). They will be hungry again, so feed them either breast milk or formula. (Don't forget to change them before they feed.)

11:30 a.m.—Daily Outing

You should try to leave the house every day. I would say that one of the biggest mistakes that twin parents make is isolating themselves. I know that it's such a project to go outside that sometimes it doesn't feel like it's even worth it, but it really is important to feel like you are a part of society and to give your day some structure. This is a good time of day to do it. It's the warmest time of the day, so in the middle of winter, this is as good as it's going to get. It doesn't matter what you do during this time. Run your errands, go to the park, or even just go for a walk with the twins in their stroller. Just get out of the house and get some fresh air with your duo.

You will need a stocked diaper bag for this outing. Please see my complete list of what to keep in your diaper bag at the end of this chapter, on page 194.

12:30 p.m.—Snack

Depending on their age, the twins might have a small breast- or bottle-feeding, or else they will have a snack. Don't forget to eat lunch yourself, too! It's fun to do this picnic style in the park during the warm seasons.

1 p.m.—Afternoon Nap

You'll want to be back home from your outing by 12:45, to get the twins ready for their second nap. You must do everything exactly the same way that you did it for the morning nap. I don't care if your kid is a newborn or a teenager—if you aren't consistent, you will not have as much success. This is the one thing that I know for sure. If you tell your kids that they won't get a treat if they don't eat their vegetables and then give in just once, they will know this is possible and will try to do it again and again. Consistency is the key, now and forever. The same thing goes for sleep training. Swaddle them if they prefer it, keep the room dark, turn on the white noise, and go.

3 p.m.—Feeding/Witching Hour

Again, no matter how long they slept, you will go in and get the twins after two hours and feed them with the breast or bottle. Then watch out, because this is the witching hour and the twins will be at their grumpiest. Remember when I said that you'd have plenty of time later to hold and cuddle them? Well, now is the time. Aren't you excited? Try to entertain them as well as you can until it's time to get them ready for bed. Feel free to start their baths early if you run out of ideas, especially if you'll be flying solo at bedtime.

6 p.m.–7 p.m.—Bedtime Routine

You can decide what routine is best for your family, but many baby bedtime routines normally start with a bath. The most important thing I can say about bathing twins is to bathe them in the sink. It's easier on your back (since you are standing) and it forces you to do your dishes or to at least stick them in the dishwasher. Again, you should only bathe one baby at a time, so if you are alone at bath time, one baby will have to wait in the baby swing or bouncy seat while the other is bathed. Just make sure that she is strapped in someplace safe so that you can focus all of your attention on the slippery, wet baby. Make sure to have two of these "home bases" for the babies so that you also have somewhere to put each one after they get out of the tub. (For more tips on bath time see pages 140–142.)

If your spouse is home or you have other help around, this is a great time to divide and conquer, meaning that you each take responsibility for one baby from bath time all the way up until they go to bed. It's a great way to spend some quality time with just one baby for a change, and then the next night you can switch babies.

After they're bathed, get the babies in their pajamas and complete the rest of your nighttime routine. Get creative and come up with a routine that will take them all the way to preschool. Go ahead and read a bedtime story, say prayers, or talk about your day. It may seem kind of ridiculous to do this kind of stuff now, but starting a routine will serve you all well into the future. This routine will include a bottle or breast-feed for now. Then you swaddle the babies and put them in their cribs for the night at 7 p.m. or earlier. If you see your babies are having trouble settling down to sleep, try moving their bedtime up a few minutes. Sound odd? They may be overtired and it's making it harder for them to fall asleep.

11 p.m.—Dream Feed

Sorry, did you think that you were done for the night? Almost. You do need to feed them one more time before you go to bed. This feeding actually doesn't have to be done at 11. If you go to bed at 10, feed them then. If you go to bed at midnight, feed them then. The point is to give them one more feeding so that they can sleep through the rest of the night—and so can you! Keep this feeding very low-key. Do not turn on the light and do not even make eye contact. Just softly pick up the babies, change them, and feed them. Try feeding them one at a time instead of together. They probably won't even wake up all the way. This is a good feeding for your spouse to do with bottles, which will let you go to sleep earlier and prevent the twins from smelling you in the room and getting all excited. Then that's it! You made it through the day. If you hear the babies cry during the night, you can leave them alone to self-soothe or else try to give them a pacifier, but once your pediatrician says it's okay, they should be able to go until morning without being fed.

If you have trouble sticking to this schedule or can't stand hearing your babies cry for more than five minutes, I understand. But before you throw in the towel, remember that the crying is a very temporary means to an end. If you follow this schedule, there should be no more crying after four days. That is a very short time in the long run when compared to months (or years) of sleepless nights for your entire family. But if this isn't for you, then simply don't do it. Never go against your instincts when it comes to your children.

If you do end up getting your children on a sleep schedule, you'll notice as they get bigger their sleeping patterns will change. A newborn requires up to sixteen hours of sleep a day and that doesn't really drop much during the first year. As they get bigger, you'll be able to adjust their sleeping schedules with a little guidance from your pediatrician. Always consult with them to see if your twins are getting enough zzzzz's.

Sleep training is a difficult time in a new mom's life. While we know it's better for them to sleep, it's hard to hear them cry. This is where husbands play a huge role. Dads are often able to tolerate the crying much more than moms are. When dads hear the babies cry, sure, they feel bad, but they can handle it. For a new mom, sirens start going off in our head, our heart starts to race, our boobs start to throb, and it's occasionally a

From the MOM Squad: *"Some days things won't work and that's okay. Switch it up until you figure out how things work best for you and the babies."* —Ericka C.

much different experience for us. DADS, LISTEN UP! Take one for the team and help us out, come sleep-training time. We need you!

Making Your Twins' Schedule Work for You

As time goes by and the twins are doing well on their schedule and sleeping through the night, you will be able to go off schedule from time to time and find ways to build flexibility into your routine. Stick to a schedule religiously while you are in the heat of sleep training, but then take each day as it comes and use the schedule as more of a guide. If it's a brutal winter and you can't get outside each day, it will be fine. If you must take the twins out during their nap time because of a special occasion, it's okay. Never forget that this schedule was designed to help you, so if it begins to feel like a prison, you need to adjust it until it better suits your life.

Don't ever forget to make room in your schedule for all of the things that you need to get done in a day, too. Believe it or not, in the beginning, you will actually have to plan on when you are going to take a shower and when you are going to go to the bathroom! For a while, you won't be able to live spontaneously and still get anything done, so you need to schedule in your personal life, too. This goes for spending time with your friends, having a cup of coffee, reading a book, and, yes, having sex with your husband. Look at the twins' daily schedule and add times for doing things for yourself. Trust me. If you don't make these things a priority, they might never happen, but if you are diligent about planning and sticking to your plan, you will be able to get everything done eventually. In the meantime, here are a few tips to help you make the most of your "free" time.

Become a Swifter Picker Upper

Try to keep your house as organized as possible so that when it's time to put away the books and toys, it's easy to do. For example, bringing all of the toys from the babies' room to the living room so they can play will make it harder to clean up when they're done. Instead, keep one basket of toys in the living room, one in the bedroom, and one anywhere else they might be playing throughout the day.

Write It Down

Whether or not you made them before you had twins, lists are now going to be your best friend. Make a list of everything that you need to do—for the children, for yourself, and for your spouse. At the end of the day, review what you've done. This is a great way to stay organized and to feel like you actually accomplished something. If you're having trouble remembering where your list is, buy a magnetic notepad and put it on the refrigerator and you won't waste any time searching or compiling multiple lists!

Do It Now

Remember that saying, "Don't put off for tomorrow what you can do today"? Well, let's take it one step further and say, "Don't put off for tomorrow morning what you can do tonight." After the twins are in bed is a great time to pack your diaper bag, wash bottles, and prepare new ones for the next day. If possible, get as much of tomorrow's work done today.

Find a Home for It

As soon as you bring something new into your home, find a home for it. If you let things stack up on your kitchen counter or anyplace else, the mess will quickly get out of hand and it will take you more time to sort through the giant pile than it would have to put away one simple item in the first place.

Pediatrician Pointers

In addition to keeping you organized, your Twins Daily logs, in Appendix B of this book, are important to your pediatrician. They are a great resource when you are discussing your twins' health. Example: if your babies aren't gaining enough weight, you'll be able to refer to the chart to see exactly how much they are drinking/eating.

During these visits it can be extremely challenging to handle two babies at the same time. Part of the problem is that occasionally pediatricians' offices will book one appointment slot for your twins as opposed to two separate appointments. This isn't really fair, is it? Of course you'll still be charged two copayments! Such is life with twins.

When scheduling appointments, if you can actually get two separate appointments, that is definitely the way to go. True, it's more time consuming but it will give you time to focus on each baby individually and you won't have to scramble to hold, change, weigh, measure, and comfort two babies at once! If you have to settle for one appointment, make sure that someone goes with you, whether it's your spouse, nanny, or mom. With two adults and two babies, you can focus exclusively on the baby in your arms. This is more challenging than it seems. It's incredibly difficult to resist comparing babies, whether they're boy/girl fraternal twins, same-sex fraternals, or identical twins. But try very hard to focus for a minute. Talk to the doctor about Baby A first, and then move on to Baby B. If you ping-pong back and forth, everyone will get confused and nothing will be accomplished. When did Baby A start sleeping through the night? How much does Baby A drink and poop? Don't say, "Well, Baby A just started sleeping through the night, but Baby B still wakes up twice to nurse." See how confusing that is?

Bring your daily charts with you and stay on the chart of the baby you're focusing on. On the chart for each baby, write down questions that pertain only to that baby. Wait until you are completely finished with Baby A, and then hand him off to your partner and focus on Baby B. Don't expect to remember your questions or the doctor's answers. Just like with the OB appointment, think about recording your session with the pediatrician or else writing everything down.

If you end up doing both appointments at once, I suggest that the vaccines be given to both babies at the exact same time. Babies have two types of cries—the everyday cry and "the house is on fire" cry. Twins will almost never react to their twin's everyday cry, but they sure will respond to the other one. This is the cry that you hear when your baby gets a shot. The baby who's just gotten the vaccine will cry like the house is on fire, and their twin will cry in response before he or she has even gotten the shot! If they get their shots at the same time, they'll both cry, but it will all be over a lot faster. To this day, if I don't give my twins their shots at the exact same time, the other one will cry. I think this is just one of those twin things that the rest of us will never fully understand. If there aren't two docs on hand to make this happen, a doctor and one of the nurses can usually handle the task.

TWINIVERSITY TIP

This is a minor tip, but it will save you a few minutes, and you'll need all the free time that you can possibly get! When you fill out pediatrician forms for your children, fill the form out once with everything except the child's name, then make a photocopy and fill in each of their names on the forms. Do not start writing two forms for every single thing. All of the information on the forms will be the same except for their names! (You can do this for school and camp forms later on, too.)

What's in Your Diaper Bag?

Like the Girl Scouts, the motto for all twin mamas *should* be "Be prepared." Any mom of multiples can tell you that preparation and planning your day can make all the difference between chaos and calmness. To help you on your way to multiple parenting successes, I've organized a list of what your diaper bag should contain so you too can "Be prepared."

Your daily diaper bag should contain:

___One diaper for every two hours per baby that you will be out (plus four extra just in case)

____ Baby wipes in a closed bag (Kirkland/Costco makes the best portable wipes)

____ At least one set of clothing for each baby in a ziplock bag (in case of a liquid spill)

____ Changing pad (disposable or reusable)

____ Diaper cream (get a travel size just for your diaper bag)

____ A few garbage bags (the small bags for dog poop are fantastic for this)

____ Extra shirt for you! (We always forget about us.)

____ Blanket for each baby

____ Hat (sunscreen, too, if babies are over six months)

____ Bottle for each child (formula- or powder-filled). If you're using powder, keep an extra serving in a ziplock bag just in case.

____ Extra breast pads (if you're breast-feeding), in case you start leaking

____ Burp cloths/bibs

____ Pacifiers, plus one or two spares (On the Go Pacifier Wipes from One Step Ahead wouldn't be such a bad idea, either)

____ Enough baby food for one and a half servings, plus a baby spoon First aid kit (antibiotic spray, Band-Aids, packet of Advil for you, twenty dollars and insurance card copies for you and the twins, along with emergency phone numbers in case of a true emergency)

____ Hand sanitizer and more hand sanitizer (go organic so you don't have to worry about the babies putting their hands in their mouths)

____ A few toys for the road!

____ Snack for yourself

____ A bottle of water or two

Yes, I know, this seems like a lot for one diaper bag but remember, you do have two babies! Also, when shopping for your diaper bag, you don't *always* have to go the conventional route. A messenger bag works just as well as a traditional diaper bag. Anything you can sling over your shoulder will do the trick so you can always remain hands-free for your kiddos.

Now if you are an overachieving mom like me, and want to go the extra mile, take note and stock your trunk or undercarriage of your stroller with all of the above, plus an assigned ziplock bag for each child containing:

___ Set of clothing*
___ Diaper
___ Wipes (again in a separate bag)

Also, the bottom of your stroller should contain:

___ Your rain cover (don't just take it out if you think you need it)
___ Poncho for you (how can you push a stroller *and* hold an umbrella?)
___ Pump to fill a flat (if you have air-filled tires on your stroller)

Now you are ready to hit the road. For more information on travel, check out chapter 11.

Remember to change the size of their clothing as they grow.

CHAPTER 10

somebody please help me

YOU'VE PROBABLY ALREADY NOTICED THAT WHENEVER YOU TELL people that you're pregnant with twins, they are very likely to say something along the lines of, "Well, I certainly hope you'll have help." Let's assume that they mean well and that they're not saying that they have no faith that you would be able to raise these children alone. In any case, I certainly do hope you have help—not because you won't be able to do it otherwise, but because it will be much harder on you if you do.

But it's easy to say that you'll have help or assume that you'll have help or just nod appreciatively whenever friends and family members tell you that they will, in fact, help. It's much more difficult to turn these abstract offers of help into actual help that is truly helpful. Hiring paid help, in the form of a nanny, babysitter, day care, or baby nurse, can be even more confusing and overwhelming. Don't worry, because this chapter is going to help you sort out every type of help imaginable and show you how to get the most out of each and every one. Soon, you'll be almost rested and nearly relaxed, thanks to all of the help you're getting.

The Friends and Family Plan

We've already discussed how to get the most help possible out of your family members and friends during the first few weeks and months of your twins' lives. Some mothers of twins are then able to keep their mother, sister, or mother-in-law on board as a full-time caretaker for their twins if and when they return to work. This seems to be becoming more and more common as grandmas are often right around retirement age when their daughters or daughters-in-law give birth, but are still young and spry enough to spend their time caring for little ones.

Whether it's full-time or just a few hours a week, having a family member as a long-term caretaker is fraught with benefits and possible downsides. Before you jump into this type of setup, take some time to think about your relationship with your mother (or mother-in-law) and how it might be affected by having her as your nanny. Will she drive you nuts? Will it bring you closer and help you create an even stronger bond or cause conflicts that might seriously damage your relationship? Will you love to see how your twinnies grow attached to her or will this make you feel jealous and resentful? Of course you can't predict exactly how you'll react to every situation, but it's a good idea to think this through. To help you do so, below are the top pros and cons to this child care scenario. Read these over and think them over before "hiring" a family member for this important job.

Grandma as Nanny Pros
* Grandma has complete unconditional love for your twins, which cannot be replicated with a nanny no matter how wonderful she may be.
* Your twins will learn the same family values and traditions that only another family member can teach.
* You may feel more comfortable leaving your twins with someone you know and trust.
* Grandma might be paid in hugs and kisses instead of actual money. Of course, this can be a huge financial benefit for your family.

- Your twins will develop a strong bond with the family member who cares for them that wouldn't be formed otherwise.
- If the kids are sick, you won't have to miss work.
- If you are sick, you'll have someone to take care of you, too!
- You can ask for things that you might not be comfortable asking a stranger to do—laundry, meal preparation, straightening up, staying late, et cetera.

Grandma as Nanny Cons

- Guilt is more of a concern than it would be with hired help. When they are stressed, you might feel bad for making them work so hard, while with a hired nanny you would view them as a professional who could handle it. Your family member might also want to go the extra mile to help you out, which might only make you feel worse.
- You might feel like you're missing out on precious time with your twins more than you would with hired help. If Grandma goes on and on about every little thing they do and how cute the twins are, you may feel even worse for missing all of that special time with them.
- Boundaries might be an issue. Do you really want your family member in your personal space every day? How might you feel having her so involved in every aspect of your life? Some grandmas may react to this situation by pushing even more and it may be next to impossible for you to create any boundaries at all.
- If your mom is watching the kids full-time, you may not feel like you can ask her to watch the kids for a date night. Having family around is a nice perk, but if your family is your sole sitter, you may have no one else to call!
- More often than not, they will spoil the kids. Yes, they may be acting as a nanny, but they are a grandparent first. It may be very tough to get your mother or mother-in-law to strictly follow your house rules.
- Your mother may have the unique ability to push all of your buttons at once. Add two babies to the mix and this could be a bad situation.

> **Note from Dad:**   *"Get rid of pride. If you need help, and you will, ask!"* —Trevor M.

Conflict on the Home Front

If your family member becomes your nanny or your babysitter, it's important to come up with a strategy for how to handle small disagreements you might have about caring for the babies or similar issues that come up. Little critiques or suggestions that might be easy to say to a nanny may feel like explosives that need to be handled extremely delicately with your mother. Of course, all of this depends on your relationship with her. Some of you might have an easier time talking to your mother-in-law than someone you hired, but if your family is on the defensive side, these situations can be very tricky. You don't want to cause any sort of rift in your family, but you do want (and deserve) to have a say in how things are handled when you're not at home.

Before talking to your mother or mother-in-law about a concern you have, make sure that your spouse is on board—especially if the situation involves your mother-in-law. Ask him what he thinks is the best way to handle the situation. Perhaps you can avoid conflict altogether and he can take one for the team by addressing it with her. (Don't count on it.) In any case, you and your spouse must always remain a united front on these issues. Remember—united we stand, divided we fall. Make sure that your husband has your back as things come up, and vice versa! Relationships between spouses can really suffer when one won't back the other one up to a family member.

Ultimately, honesty is really the best policy here, as it so often is. If you fail to address issues that come up, your feelings of resentment might grow and damage the relationship with your mother or mother-in-law even more. Just talk things out as they come up in a light, breezy manner, and try to steer clear of judgmental or critical tones. Don't forget to thank your

From the MOM Squad: *"Get a network of support in place before your wee ones arrive. Friends, family, etc. to help with errands, laundry, watching babies so you can sleep or shower . . . that way you can concentrate on taking care of yourself and your babies." —Michele H.*

family member for the wonderful service that she is doing for your family, even when she's not doing it perfectly. Just expressing your gratitude can help smooth these things over more than anything else.

Calling in the Pros

If you prefer to hire a professional to care for your little ones or don't have any other option, there are many different types of paid help out there who are ready and willing to care for your twins. Here is a breakdown of the different types of professional help you can hire, a ballpark figure of how much they cost, and what you can expect to get from them.

Baby Nurse

A baby nurse comes to your home to care for your twins for a twenty-four-hour period anywhere from three to seven days a week. Most baby nurses won't actually work seven days a week, plus you should remember that most of them have families of their own that they should be able to see every so often. The downside, of course, is that baby nurses are pricey. In New York City they charge up to $350 a night. While she's there, a baby nurse will change, settle, and feed (if you're bottle-feeding) the babies. She might even do the babies' laundry and wash the bottles after the babies eat.

Baby nurses are usually hired on a very temporary basis—to get you through those first few weeks with the twins. If you fall in love with your baby nurse and she decides that she wants to stay with you, she can sometimes transition into a nanny, but she would have to take a huge pay cut to do that, so don't count on that happening. We did have one Twiniversity member who kept her baby nurse for three years, but she obviously had Rockefeller money. If you can do that, go for it. I'm just jealous.

Because your baby nurse will likely only be with you for a few nights or weeks, it is very important for you to get as much help as you can from her. Don't just sit there and think, "I'm paying her $350 a night. I'm just going to sit here, eat this grilled cheese, and watch TV." That's not doing you any service. You might be resting and recovering from your delivery, but you need to use that baby nurse like she's a teacher. Watch everything that she does, and say, "How did you do that? What can I do better?"

However, I will tell you that 50 percent of baby nurses are going to want you to leave them alone to do things their way and just bring you the babies when it's time to nurse. The other half of baby nurses, though, are going to be really excited to help you. This is something to look for when you're interviewing baby nurses. If you go through an agency, tell them that you're looking for someone who is interested in teaching you things. Otherwise, make it clear during the interview so that you'll find someone who is truly willing to educate you, or at least who can't act like you didn't warn her.

Night Nurse

Night nurses do the same things as baby nurses, except that they're only there for a twelve-hour period at night—usually from 7 p.m. to 7 a.m., for example. A night nurse costs almost or close to exactly the same amount as a regular baby nurse.

So why would you pay the same amount for only half the hours? Well, one reason is space. If you hate having people in your home or you don't have the extra room for somebody, then you get the night nurse and nobody's underfoot for those extra twelve hours while you're awake. I say, if you have the space, go for the baby nurse and get as much as you can from her while she's there.

Postpartum Doula

A birth doula's job is to support a laboring woman through birth, and a postpartum doula is there to support the new mother after the birth. Basically, a postpartum doula is a new mother's lady-in-waiting. The main difference between a doula and a baby nurse is that the baby nurse is just there for the twins, while a doula is there for you and the twins. She usually will cook for you, clean for you, care for the babies, and do basically anything else that you want or need her to do. She is there to educate you, to make sure that you are a whole person, and check that you're healing properly. Doulas will help with breast-feeding, and many postpartum doulas are actually certified lactation consultants. Basically, it's a very organic, nurturing experience for both the mother and babies.

The cost of a doula can range anywhere from fifteen to seventy-five dollars an hour and higher, based on their experience and certifications. Besides asking everyone you know, the best way to find a doula is to go to the national organization's website, www.dona.org.

Au Pairs

If you have the extra room, I think this is totally the way to go if you think you will need a lot of help. These are international students who basically serve as live-in nannies. They come to the U.S.A. on a one- or two-year visa. That's the downside—you only have them for a short amount of time, so you have to train someone new each year or every other year. Au pairs are fairly inexpensive compared to the cost of a typical live-in nanny. You might pay around two hundred dollars a week for an au pair, compared to at least triple that for other live-in help.

Mother's Helper

A mother's helper is somebody who will do the miscellaneous jobs that you will no longer have time to do once the twins are born. They could pick up the dry cleaning, for example, or take the dog for a walk. They're basically your personal assistant. Or you can use a mother's helper more like a regular babysitter so that you can take a break or get some errands done. A great way to find mother's helpers is through local colleges. Call the Placement Department of a local college that has an early childhood program.

This is a great option if you're not pinned into a corner, schedule-wise, and can offer some flexibility in exchange for a lower salary. Of course, most mother's helpers won't have the same experience as someone who's been a baby nurse for twenty-five years, but they'll be excited to come play with your twins, plus you're going to pay them! You can usually get away with paying a college student about eight to ten dollars an hour, and if you throw in your leftovers from last night, they'll be superexcited.

Nanny

I saved nannies for last because you usually hire them later on, when you're thinking about going back to work or once you have an established schedule and know when you're going to need to fill in holes with care for your twins. A nanny is obviously there for her shift based on whatever hours you agree on. In New York City, where I live, an average nanny will make eighteen dollars an hour (and yes, that is for twins). Outside of my fair city, Twiniversity members generally pay between eight and twenty dollars an hour, depending on where they live.

A lot of people ask me how important it is that their nanny has twin experience. I actually don't think it's that important. It's much more essential to find somebody who fits in with your family. Plus, my big issue with nannies who have lots of twin experience is that not all of their tricks are good. Sure, they might have figured out how to feed two babies in one arm, but that's not a great idea, even if they have been doing it for thirty years. If you have somebody who just clicks with your family, it will all work out better in the long run. Now, if they have worked for one or two twin families, that's a bonus, but in my opinion it ranks as maybe a four or a five on the priority list.

Ten Tips for Hiring Help

Now that you know which kinds of help are available, I'm going to walk you through the process of finding and hiring the right help for you. As for timing, I recommend starting the hiring process about two months before you want this person to begin. You want to interview night nurses while you're still pregnant, for example. And you'll want to look for nannies two months before the end of your maternity leave and ask them to start at least two weeks before you're set to go back to work so that you have that time together to get comfortable. Many moms find this entire process overwhelming and awkward, especially if they've never hired any type of household help before, but with these ten steps to hiring help, you'll feel like a pro.

Tip 1: Consider an Agency

Yes, it costs more, but I believe that going through an agency to hire a babysitter or nanny is best. Why? First of all, they do all of the work for you. Plus, they have built-in referrals. For example, you can call an agency and say that you want someone who's been working with them for a minimum of two years. An agency typically does all the background checks and will have two years' worth of references. Most agencies also put their staff through some rigorous training courses, which is another bonus. If you choose to use an agency, make sure you find out what their hiring process is. Double-check to see what background and credit checks they do just to give yourself an extra dose of peace of mind.

Tip 2: Get Descriptive

If you decide to hire directly instead, you're going to have to sit down and write out a job description. You can just make a list of everything that you want this person to do and when you want them to do it. That includes the schedule, the tasks, the pay, and the bonuses. Are you going to pay them on the books or off? Are you going to give them gas money or let them use your car? Are you going to buy them a cell phone? Write it all out in as much detail as possible. It's very realistic for you to expect your nanny to:

- Take care of the children's clothing (washing, sorting, folding, putting away all of their stuff). They can even choose the outfits for the children when they are not on duty.
- Take care of your children's meals. They can prepare breakfast (either the day of, or day before), lunch, and dinner for your children.
- They should attend all classes and activities that you have set up for your children during their typical work hours and also provide safe transportation to and from.
- They should be a positive role model for your kiddos. They should be loving, nurturing, and be able to keep your children safe and happy.

Tip 3: Post It

Post your job description in several places, including your local twins club bulletin board, Craigslist, and any other local moms' sites you can think of. Also, e-mail it to your neighborhood parenting, church, and community groups, and everyone you know, asking them if they know anyone who might fit the bill.

Tip 4: Create an Application

This might sound nutty, but create a job application. You need a simple form with the following questions: their name, legal name, address, past addresses, phone numbers, references, and Social Security number. You might want to consider conducting a background check, in which case you have to let them know that you will be doing this. (You can even put this in the job description.) If you do, you'll already have all the information you need.

TWINIVERSITY TIP

Are your nanny's vaccines up to date? Make sure she has all her current shots. Adults need vaccines, too.

Tip 5: Take Pictures of Each Applicant

When it's time to interview applicants, snap a picture of each person on your cell phone. Again, this might sound crazy, but if you are interviewing eight people in one day you probably will not remember who Tina was unless you have a picture of her. Then make sure you write down all of their answers. Whether you're going through this process before or after the twins are born, you're probably not getting any sleep and won't remember anything unless you write it down!

Tip 6: Have Your Questions Ready and Let Your Interviewee Talk

When it's time to interview, have your list of questions ready and ask the exact same questions to every person you are going to interview. You may love Angela's answer to a certain question and hire her for that reason, but what if Jenny had an even better answer but you neglected to ask? Don't forget to write down their answers, too. I promise you won't remember what everyone said. A complete list of suggested interview questions appears below.

Try not to talk too much. Just ask questions and let the applicant answer freely. The more information they willingly give the better. You don't want to guide the candidate indirectly by saying things like, "You can stay late on Thursdays, right?" Don't jump to conclusions.

Nanny Interview Questions
- Why did you become a nanny?
- How often do you plan to meet your friends for "playdates" during working hours?
- How much time do you need to spend on your cell phone during working hours?
- When do you expect a pay raise?
- What do you do when you go to the park/playgroup with the kids?

- Are you prepared to fill out a form for us to carry out a background check?
- Are there prior/current jobs, and how/when/why did the job relationship end?
- What would be a typical day with my children?
- How do you deal with temper tantrums/how do you discipline children?
- Has a parent ever asked you to do something you disagreed with or have you ever disagreed with how a parent handled their child? If so, how did you deal with it?
- What will it be like for you to be there while I work from home?
- Do you have any health issues that might interfere with your job?
- What kind of activities will you do with my babies?
- How do you handle an emergency? Are you trained in CPR?
- What do you like about being a nanny? What don't you like?
- How would you get to work every day?
- If they have kids of their own: What are your backup child care options?
- Are you willing to come early or stay late (for extra pay), if needed?

Tip 7: Cover the Basics (and the Not-So-Basics)

The most important points to cover are the work schedule, salary, taxes, overtime, benefits (whether you're going to actually give medical benefits or little things like a bus pass and a cell phone), and vacation. Typically, you give two weeks of vacation for full-time help: one week that you choose and one week that they choose, but this can vary from family to family. You want to talk about raises and bonuses. For example, you might want to start out with a low salary and say that you'll do a review in three months and give a raise then based on performance.

Many parents forget to talk about phone usage and TV viewing. Here's the deal—if you don't tell your nanny that you don't want them on the phone, who's to say that she's not going to be on her cell all the time? True story—I can't even count the number of nannies I've seen with a Bluetooth headset talking on the phone for two and a half hours while I was at the playground with my own twins. If you don't want that to happen, you need to say, "I don't feel comfortable with your being on the phone while the children are awake." If you don't say this and then you find out that your nanny was on the phone all day, you'll have no right to complain. The same thing goes for the TV. If you don't want them watching *Judge Judy*, you need to say that. If it doesn't bother you, that's fine, but don't get mad at her for watching *Mad Men* while she bottle-feeds the twins if you never told her not to.

Tip 8: Always Check References

Don't rely on one source as your reference. Call several people. This is where another parent of twins would come in handy, because a twin parent will be very honest when talking to another parent of twins. As twin parents, we sometimes shelter our singleton friends a little bit by sugarcoating things, but we save the cold hard truth for each other.

Tip 9: Keep It Legal

You should *not* hire a nanny who does *not* have the legal right to work in this country. This way, if they get hurt, God forbid, they're entitled to disability insurance. They'll get Social Security benefits, as well.

Tip 10: Hire Everyone!

Once you've done all of this, if you've found a few people you like, I strongly suggest that you hire a few of them. Sound crazy? You hire them each for one day. The truth is that no matter how many questions you ask, you have no idea what they're going to be like until they're actually there. They may have an allergy to cats that you never thought to ask about, and now they're in your house and they're sneezing all over the place from your kitty. So hire every nanny whom you like for a day and see how you feel once they've all done a day's work. Have them meet the kids and see what they're like. Stay home, then go out for a little bit, or buy a nanny cam and watch it the whole time.

Day Care

The other common form of child care for your twins is obviously day care. You can't (and shouldn't and, hopefully, wouldn't) put your twins in day care until they are at least six weeks old, so you'll be choosing between day care and a nanny or between day care and staying at home with your twins, not between day care and a night nurse or a postpartum doula. Day care centers are basically facilities that are certified to care for several children at once. They are normally quite expensive, but so are nannies. If you were having a single child, day care might be the more affordable option. However, the same isn't necessarily true for twins. Sending two children to day care will cost double the amount of sending one, while a nanny may only charge a bit more per hour for the second child.

Some offices have on-site day care, which to me justifies this additional expense. If your office has a day care, you can drop in on the twins all day and even stop by to nurse them if you want.

Another big pro of day care is that it has structured activities, so your twins will be fluent in Mandarin before they are two, and they will go on field trips to museums and zoos. On the other hand, the con to day care is that the fourteen other children there are like carrier monkeys, and could potentially give your kids every sickness under the sun in their first year. Pediatricians say that this isn't bad, because the more they are sick when they are little, the less they'll be sick when they're big. Try telling that to a mother of sick six-month-old twins, though.

The other issue with day care for twins is that we lucky parents of twins have to fight for two slots. This can be a big problem in a big city where there is a lot of demand for day care. I hate to say it, but this is an even bigger issue if you have identical twins or same-sex twins, because schools try to balance out the classes and you'll be taking up two boy slots or two girl slots.

Nanny vs. Day Care vs. Staying at Home

Before we move on from the topic of help, I want to talk about the option of staying home from work instead of hiring a nanny or sending the twins to day care. Before making this decision, you need to figure out exactly what you're making in a year—and I don't just mean what it says on your pay stub. How much are you spending on clothing, commuting, and any additional expenses? Compare that to how much you'll really be paying your day care or nanny, including anything above and beyond a flat salary, from health insurance to a cell phone. When it all shakes out, you may realize that you're really only making two thousand dollars a year.

You have to decide for yourself what makes it worth it. Now, some people just don't want to be stay-at-home parents or can't because even after you look at the bottom line, the benefits at your job are too good to be true, and that is fine. In this case, you should go back to work even if you're only breaking even. But if you've always toyed with the idea of staying at home, figure out what your bottom line is and see if it makes sense. With the additional cost of child care, twin mamas are more likely to decide to stay at home when the babies are little, and I personally think that's a great choice if you can swing it. Here are some of the top pros and cons to nannies, day cares, and staying at home to help guide you toward making the right decision for your family.

Nanny Pros

Cost-Effective

At an average of twelve to fifteen dollars an hour for twins, nannies are definitely more affordable for twins than most day cares.

Sick Kids = No Sweat

You can't (and shouldn't) send a sick baby to day care, and parents often scramble for backup care when one of their kids is sick. Multiply this times two and you get a lot of headaches, especially during your babies' first year. With a nanny, however, you don't need a backup option because she is set to work even when the kids are sick.

Customizable

Your nanny should follow your specific instructions and the rules that you set just for your kids. Your twins will be fed when and where you want them to be and should be taken care of exactly how you prefer. This would obviously be impossible at a busy day care facility.

Flexibility

You set your nanny's schedule, so you can make sure that it works with your vacation time, commute, et cetera. Day cares have set daily schedules and vacations that may not match up with your preferences.

There's No Place Like Home

You can rest assured that your kids are being cared for in the comfort of their own home, sleeping in their own cribs, and playing with all of the wonderful toys and gear that you bought specifically for them. This is a huge psychological benefit, especially for twin moms like me who tend to feel guilty.

Nanny Cons

Background Check

You might not be able to do a full background check of your nanny, especially if she hasn't lived in this country for long. This may make you feel a bit ill at ease leaving your children in her care.

Stability

You can't be completely sure how committed your nanny is to your family, especially at first.

What's stopping her from taking a better offer and forcing you to go through the laborious hiring process all over again?

Expensive Perks

Your nanny may come with additional expenses that really add up, such as a cell phone, bus or transportation money, meals, and so on. When these are taken into account, the nanny may not seem so cost-effective after all.

The Stress of Finding the Right Fit

It can be difficult to find the perfect nanny for your family. The hiring process might take a long time and could become very stressful if you haven't found the right person and you are planning to go back to work. It's a big decision and it can be difficult to find someone you trust right away.

Backup Required

You still need backup care when the nanny herself is sick (or if her children are sick) or unable to come to work one day.

Day Care Pros

Babysitting Plus

Day cares offer more than just babysitting. Your twins will also be learning and exploring new things every day that would be impossible with a nanny or stay-at-home mom. Are you ready to teach the babies yoga? A day care might be.

Social Life

In day care, your twins will be playing with other kids every day and will learn from those other kids, too. Day care kids are often more socially advanced than their peers.

Privacy Is the Best Policy

You don't have to deal with having someone in your home every day. This is a huge advantage if you are a private person or like your personal space.

Day Care Cons

The Price Is Not Right

Depending on where you live, day care for two babies can be quite expensive. Unfortunately, I've never heard of a day care offering a two-for-one deal!

Sick Days

A twin who is sick has to stay home, and you have to either stay home, too, or find some other form of child care. With two kids, this could add up to you taking a lot of vacation days that will feel like anything but vacation.

Wait Lists

In many metro areas like New York City, popular day cares have long wait lists. Sometimes you have to even put your twins on a wait list before they're born! (I wish I were kidding.) This is a problem if you want to wait a while before deciding whether to return to work.

Picking Up Bad Habits

Learning from other kids is a pro, but it's also a con when your twins are educated in how to hit, bite, or pick their noses! There's nothing like other kids to teach your angelic twins some really bad habits.

Not as Much Personal Attention

It would be impossible for a day care to give your twins the same attention that you or a full-time caregiver would. They just don't have the manpower to rock your twins to sleep, sing to them lovingly while feeding them a bottle, and so on. You will have to get used to the idea of your twins getting a little less one-on-one time during the day.

The Germ Factor

There's no question that kids in day care get sick far more often than their peers, especially during their first year. With twins, this is even more of an issue because your two little ones will give each other any germs they pick up in day care.

Pros for Staying at Home

Security Solved

With your loving eyes on your twins all day, you'll have no doubts about their safety and security. If one of the twins has a bruise, you'll know exactly how it got there. And you never have to question whether or not your rules are being followed.

You Know Their Routine

You'll know exactly what your twins are eating and drinking, when they sleep, et cetera. It will be easier for you to track any allergies or food reactions when you feed the twins every meal yourself, know right away if they seem to be getting sick, and so forth.

No Pickups and Drop-offs

Forget about the harried commutes to pick the twins up from day care or to relieve your nanny. When you are a stay-at-home mom, your schedule is at your complete discretion and your time doesn't belong to anyone else (except your two tiny new bosses, of course).

Being There for the Big Moments

Staying at home isn't for everyone (see cons below), but there is no replacement for being there for all of your twins' first moments. No one you hire can give your twins the exact same mothering love that you can, and you'll never miss an exciting moment if you choose to stay at home to care for your twins.

Cons for Staying at Home

Boredom

It's hard to imagine being bored when you're so busy caring for two infants, but stay-at-home moms do often get bored by completing the same repetitive, often thankless tasks day in and day out.

No Breaks

When you stay at home with your twins, you don't get one minute "off the clock." Your twins are there when you wake up, there all day, and there when you go to sleep. And then they're still there the next day! This can be suffocating for some moms.

No Sick Days

Being a stay-at-home mom isn't a job that you can call in sick for! If you get sick, which is pretty likely with two babies, you'll have to arrange some sort of backup care or find the strength to get through the day regardless.

Financial Hit

If you were working before the twins were born, it will be a big financial hit for your family for you to stay at home. Crunch those numbers and see if you can afford to stop working, even temporarily.

Losing Ground

If you spent your entire life building your career before twins, depending on your job, you may have a hard time reentering the workplace when you do decide to hit the pavement again.

It's Hard!

Taking care of not one but two babies is incredibly challenging, both physically and emotionally. Your babies' constant need for your love, attention, loving arms, and breast milk (if you're nursing) can be draining.

From the MOM Squad: "My husband and I finally decided that our careers were in place, so it was time to start a family. I estimated the cost of day care and diapers and knew I wanted to breast-feed. We had excellent health insurance, so that would not be a problem. We knew we would be able to afford it with no problem! Then at seven weeks we found out it was twins. We doubled the cost of day care and diapers, then figured in the cost of second car seats, cribs, high chairs, etc., and finally we discovered it would take three weeks of my salary to pay for one month of baby needs. I decided that one week of pay wasn't worth someone else raising my kids, so I became a stay-at-home mom on a tight budget . . . which became an even tighter budget when I couldn't produce milk and had to start buying formula! It has been a struggle, but worth every penny! They are three now and I am back to work part-time." —Heidi W.

Back to Work

If you do decide to return to work after the twins are born, you'll have a whole host of new issues to deal with—from the joys of finding an appropriate place in the office to pump to the stress of double day care drop-offs and commuting. This stress doesn't just apply to Mom, either. Many people forget that the transition from paternity leave to full-time work can also be very difficult and upsetting for new dads. Here are some tips and tricks to get you on your way to a successful transition.

Start Slow

Have your twins' caregiver start a few weeks before the actual date you're supposed to be back at work. Once they know your twins' daily routine, start "practicing" what your regular day will look like. Have them show up at the time that they will when you're back at work and take this time to go out and run your errands, go to the movies, or go buy yourself some new clothes for work. Just get out of the house so that the children can start to experience what it's like not to have you there.

Start off slow by going out for an hour at a time, then start to stay out longer and longer. Before you know it, you'll be out for your entire workday while your caregiver is at home with the twins. Not only is this good for you and the twins, but it will give your caregiver the confidence to handle the day without calling you at work a thousand times with questions.

Eat Your Wheaties

My husband always says that he was amazed by how well he was able to function at work after the twins were born when he was getting very little sleep each night. But if you can get your twins on a schedule and sleeping through the night before your return to work, I highly recommend it (see chapter 9 for more on this). Eating a good diet is also very important during this stressful time, especially if you're nursing. Just make sure to take extra good care of yourself during this time so that you can keep up your strength and health.

Get Your Boobs Ready

If you're planning to continue nursing after going back to work, you'll need the right supplies for pumping and storing your milk. First, you'll need a very efficient breast pump and appropriately sized storage containers. When it comes to keeping your milk fresh, you'll need a few ice packs and a place to keep the milk during the day—either a minifridge for your office or a cooler of some sort. If you want to make sure to keep up your supply, it's important that you pump at the same time that you would typically be feeding the twins. Don't forget that it's also an option to nurse your twins when you're at home and supplement with formula when you're at work. This may affect your supply, so be careful with this route if it's important to you to continue nursing, but it is an option for some moms.

Let the Guilt Go

Most working mothers carry a ton of guilt for not being home with their twinnies. If you need to go back to work either to support your family or to keep your own sanity, it's okay. Your children will be fine. You'll have every evening after work, every weekend, and every morning before you go to the office to see your little monkeys grow and thrive. They will be okay. Yes, they will miss you, but they miss you when you go to the bathroom. Their experience of time is not the same as ours. What feels like a very long day to us filled with meetings, phone conferences, and lunches was just a trip to the park, some fun stories, and some art projects to them.

Skype with the Babies

If you have a moment during the day when you just need to see their tiny little faces, that's totally normal. Perhaps you should consider investing in a security camera that allows you to access the images via a secure online website, or even Skype. It will be comforting to know that at any time of the day, you can see your babies. It's also not the worst idea to keep an eye on your caregiver and see exactly what she's doing during the day. If you do, you should tell her frankly. And in general, I don't think it's the best idea—you don't want to undermine your relationship with your nanny, an important part of your family—and at the end of the day you *have* to trust her.

Warning: Don't get in trouble at work for watching your new favorite Web reality show called *The Twins*. When you need to, pop online for a quick minute or two, and then go right back to work.

CHAPTER 11

traveling with the circus

HOPE THAT I'VE ALREADY CONVINCED YOU TO TRAVEL OUT OF YOUR house each day with the twins, but going on a longer journey with them is an entirely different matter! The thought of long car trips, train rides, and even flights with infant twins may be overwhelming or even downright terrifying. It honestly doesn't have to be. Traveling with twins is possible and can be almost painless if you have the right equipment, techniques, and attitude. That said, there are some trips that just won't be worth all the schlepping and you may have to sit some of them out. In this chapter, I'll guide you through deciding which is which and help you manage the trips you choose to make with confidence.

This is probably a good time to tell you that before I had the twins, I worked in the travel industry. So trust me when I say that I have every trick you will ever need for every type of trip with your twins, from the simplest outings to transatlantic flights. From how to win over your seatmates to how to handle switching time zones and packing for twins, I've got you covered, so just sit back, relax, and try your best to enjoy the ride.

The Freak Show Element

Only parents of twins (and other multiples) can fully appreciate what it's like to be accosted by every stranger who comes across their path wanting to ask all sorts of personal questions about their babies! It could be in the grocery store or halfway across the world: people are fascinated by multiple births. Here are some of the most common questions and comments that Twiniversity families hear when they are out and about with their duo.

"Now You Don't Have to Have Any More Kids!"

When people saw that I had twins (a boy and a girl, no less), they would often say something along the lines of, "Oh good, you got it all out of the way," or, "Now you're done." Perhaps they were trying to help me find the silver lining in my twin mama status, but it really bothered me that they felt the need to get all involved in my uterus. It was just way too personal for me, especially because I knew that I couldn't have any more children. The last thing I wanted to hear was, "Well, it's good that you're all done," from someone who didn't know me from a hole in the wall. I'll admit that I had to walk away from strangers sometimes to avoid going ballistic!

"Why Don't They Look Alike?"

Folks would look at my stroller and ask, "Are they twins?" When I said yes, they would ask if they were identical, and I would say, "No. That's a boy and that's a girl." Then very often they would ask, "Why don't they look alike?" It was as if that person had never come across another set of twins who weren't identical. I wasn't asked this once or twice, but dozens and dozens of times. You gotta love strangers.

"How Are 'the Twins'?"

It really bothers some parents of twins to have their kids referred to as "the twins" instead of by their names. It is amazing how often people do this. We've even received holiday cards written out to "Natalie, John, and the twins." This never really upset me, but as your twins get older it does become more important to call them each by name instead of always grouping them together as "the twins." Your children should always know that they are individuals first and foremost, so set the example by always calling them by name. However, my children now never miss an opportunity to let strangers know that they are twins.

"Look Out—It's Double Trouble!"

Why do some people always have to find the negative in every situation? Why do people refer to twins as double trouble instead of double the pleasure? Whenever someone would say something like this to me, I would simply respond, "Well, I couldn't decide who to leave at the hospital, so I took them both home."

"Were They Conceived Naturally?"

If I had a nickel for every time somebody asked me if I conceived my twins via IVF, I would be richer than a Trump. I have no idea why strangers decide to ask such personal questions when they see a double stroller coming down the street, but you'll see that it happens a lot. Then not only do they ask if they were conceived via IVF, but they want more details. "Was it one egg that split in two?" "How many did they put in?" (You can thank Octomom for that one!) At these times, I would simply respond, "Why, are you having trouble conceiving?" Or, "Wow, that's a bit personal." Sometimes you just need to help people remember about those manners that they have lurking inside of them somewhere.

Early Outings

As hard as it is to take care of twins at home, it only gets more complicated and difficult once you leave the house. That doesn't mean that you should become a recluse during your babies' first few months! Getting out with your twins is an important skill for you to master, and over time you *will* master it and look back on the days when you were afraid to take your new entourage out of the house. The trick is to stay calm and remain realistic about how long everything will take and how much you can really get done at a time. It may take all day just to get some groceries, but it will be worth it in order for you to feel like you can accomplish something like this by yourself.

If you're really nervous about your first outing, try taking the twins out in the car to run errands that can all be done via drive-throughs. You can actually get a lot done this way—get coffee, deposit some checks, maybe even indulge in some fast food. This will get you out of the house while keeping everyone contained in their seats. Bring a book with you in case one or both babies fall asleep while you're on the road. That would be a very good bonus!

When you're ready to leave the car, pick a familiar place for your first outing—perhaps a playground, mall, or grocery store near your home. Don't travel far or expect to get too much done. Set a small goal for yourself and gradually increase those goals over time. Before long, you'll be getting all of your chores done with both babies in a snap. These short trips out of the house will give you the confidence you need to start taking longer trips down the road.

Getting Groceries

With newborn or infant twins, even something as simple as getting your weekly groceries can turn into a major production that must be strategically planned down to the minute. But groceries must be bought and you can't let your twins stop you from this basic (and frequent) errand. Here are some of my top tips for getting groceries with your new twosome.

Plan Ahead

You may have loved strolling the aisles for meal inspiration before having twins. I'm sorry, but those days are over if you bring your twins to the store with you. You will be too distracted to even notice what's on the store shelves. Don't leave the house without an exact list of everything you need so that you can grab items mindlessly while focusing on your twins— bonus points if you sort your list by aisle.

Feed Beforehand

Make sure everyone (including you!) is fed and dry before you leave the house. Check the babies' diapers again before going into the store, because the last thing you want is a poop explosion in the middle of aisle seven.

Park by Carts

It's always a good idea to park your car as close to the cart-return station as possible. This will allow you to get a cart and return it later without ever leaving the car's side (or your babies'). Leave your trunk or hatchback open as a visual clue to other drivers that you are present when loading and unloading.

Plan Your Navigation

There are a few ways to best navigate the store. Try wearing one baby in a sling and pushing the other baby in the double stroller, using the empty stroller seat and the basket underneath to hold groceries. You can also try using two carts with one baby seated in each and push one while pulling the other once they are sitting up on their own. If your babies are still in their car seats, place one car seat over the seat of the cart and one over the basket. Make sure everyone is secure. You will still have room to slide things into the basket. Please use caution with this method and secure the car seats so that they will not fall off and your groceries don't collapse on the babies.

Bring Your Own Bags

Take your own reusable grocery bags wherever you go! You can secure them onto your stroller or on the outside of your shopping cart with a stroller hook. When you go to check out, empty the items to be scanned and take the bags off to be refilled after they are scanned. **Warning:** If you load up the bags too much and they are attached to the stroller, you could tip the babies.

Ask for Help

Don't be afraid to ask for help when you need it. Ask someone to help you to your car by carrying your bags. Ask someone to get an item off a shelf for you. Ask someone to push your cart into the next aisle. Most people will be more than willing to help out someone with two adorable babies. (And if they're not, please get their address and home number for me.)

Wear Your Twins?

Baby wearing (or carrying your baby in a soft infant carrier) has been growing in popularity over the past few years, and there are more and more options now for parents who prefer to wear their babies than push them in a stroller. Experts agree that contact with a parent helps babies thrive, and baby wearing is a great way to get close to your little ones. In addition, it leaves your hands free to get things done while you're out and about.

Some parents of twins assume that baby wearing is not for them, but that is not necessarily the case. Parents of twins can take part in the baby wearing trend, either by wearing one baby and pushing the other in a stroller, wearing a baby during those rare times when you are out with just one baby, or even by wearing both babies at once! Yes, I said it. Tandem baby wearing is not very common, and is tricky to do safely, but it can and has been done.

Parents of twins praise ring slings for being the most adaptable carriers and therefore the easiest to use with twins. You can try different positions with one or both babies to find the ones that work best for you.

You can wear your babies in separate carriers—one on your back and one on your front! Twiniversity moms like soft carriers such as the Britax Baby Carrier or Ergo for the back and ring slings in the front. You can even double up and wear one carrier on the front and one on the back. It might get bulky, but hey—it's a great workout.

Baby wearing can be a big help if one or both of your babies are colicky or you need new ways of coping with their regular fussy moments. Babies are usually soothed by being carried. Carriers are also good for naps. Babies are famously put to sleep by motion, so before your twins are on a nap schedule, you can get one or both of them to sleep by putting them in a carrier and going for a walk. If only one baby is sleepy, you can get him or her to sleep on you in a carrier while you play with the wakeful baby.

Learning to use new carriers with twins can be very tricky! If you are worried, try practicing with a doll or teddy bear before attempting to wear your twins. When it's time to load up the twins, find a time when they are both fed and rested—a grumpy baby will not make this any easier. It's also a good idea to use a "spotter" the first few times you try strapping them on to make sure that everyone is strapped in properly. Always make sure that both babies in the carrier(s) have open airways and can breathe by making sure that their chins aren't curled against their chests and that their faces aren't covered, and only using carriers that are appropriate for your twins' age and size.

> **Note from Dad:** *"I think I'm 'on the go' a little more. House projects and errands take a lot longer now with at least two, sometimes three or four in tow, and of course we get stopped in the store a lot more for the 'Are they twins? You have your hands full' conversations. But I feel more blessed, filled with wonder and laughter and love at the things they all do. My friends with just one seemed to have had a change in their lives, but they also still do the same things like leagues, getaway weekends, golfing, etc. which, well, with four under five in the house, maybe someday I might get to do one or two of those things again."* —Andy K.

Trips to the Emergency Room

I've had the occasion of going to the emergency room more than twenty-five times since my twins were born seven years ago. The first visit was for nursemaid's elbow when my son was less than two years old, and since then we've gone there because of my twins' affinity for the croup. All of our trips to the ER have granted my husband and me honorary degrees in preparation for such visits. I never really thought about how good we had gotten at it until one night at the ER when I made "IcePack 3000" for my daughter to place on the spot where she had just received an injection to reduce the swelling in her larynx. It consisted of a latex glove filled with ice, attached with an Ace bandage. A nurse walked in, saw our contraption, and said, "What a great idea; I'm totally stealing that for my other patients." Coming from a nurse with over twenty years of experience, this meant a lot, and I am happy to share my ER tips with you, in hopes that you never, ever need them.

The first thing you need to do is find out if any of your local hospitals have a pediatric emergency room. You may even be lucky enough to have a dedicated children's hospital nearby. Decide (right now) which hospital you would visit in an emergency and know the route to it.

It's just as important not to overreact as it is not to underreact. Deciding when your child really needs an emergency room versus just a doctor can be really tricky. You need an ER if your child can't breathe or is unconscious, or if your child took a bad fall and is now complaining of blurry vision or a headache. These are just a few definites, but you should always trust your instincts. As a parent, Mother Nature gave you the right amount of alarm, so pay attention to it and don't delay. It's better to take an unnecessary trip to the ER than to regret not going later.

When heading to the emergency room, put on your best smile and act as enthusiastic as you can. Putting a good spin on a bad situation will keep you and the baby calm. Try to be thoughtful when deciding what your child will wear if it's not a true emergency. Put on socks and pants (for girls who might be in a nightgown if it's nighttime) and a sweater. Hospitals are cold.

In most cases, when you get to the ER you will check in and give just your name. There will be a separate desk for the rest of your information. Next, be prepared to wait. Unless your child comes in via ambulance, you will go to a room and wait to be called by the triage nurse. When called, the nurse will take your child's pulse oxygen level by putting a monitor on their finger. They will also take your child's temperature (the method varies by hospital). They might take their blood pressure as well. This will be your chance to tell them what is going on. From there, they will decide the severity of the situation and act accordingly.

If you feel the hospital is not making an appropriate choice, ask to speak to the person in charge. **Note:** Be as nice as possible. Like the old saying goes, you can catch more flies with honey than with vinegar. From triage, you will usually be taken to a room or a bed where you'll be seen by a few doctors. Depending on the issue, it could be an orthopedic (bone) doctor, a pulmonologist (lung/breathing) doctor, or someone else. You will always be seen by the resident pediatrician as well. Most important, remain calm and remember that if I've survived twenty-five ER visits, you can surely make it through this one.

Trains, Planes, and Automobiles

Whether it's a simple car trip to Grandma's house or a cross-country flight, any type of travel with young twins can be an adventure all on its own. But that doesn't mean that you have to be house (or neighborhood) bound for your twins' entire first year! Follow these tips from Twiniversity moms who have mastered the art of twin travel and the trip will be a lot less bumpy.

Before heading out on a big journey, make sure that you write down lists of all the items you'll need to bring with you for every member of the family. These lists can be anywhere—on your phone, on a notepad, or on a loose sheet of paper. Just make sure that they include everything you need and that you check them while you pack your bags. Not only will these lists come in handy when you're packing for your trip, they'll ensure that you have everything with you when it's time to come home. The lists should include things like medications, favorite toys, and even underwear and socks or a particular outfit that you want the twins to wear on the trip. This will take all of the guesswork out of packing and make your destination feel like home away from home.

One great idea to help you prepare is to call for backup the night before your big trip. Another pair of hands in the house to take care of the twins while you pack your bags will help you keep your sanity and ensure that you remember to pack everything on your lists. If you wait until after the twins go to bed to start packing, you might get too tired yourself and forget some things that you shouldn't. And be sure to remember: If you are traveling to a family member's house, send them your shopping list in advance (some money would be nice, too). That way, everything you need will be waiting for you when you arrive. It will make things so much easier if you have formula, diapers, et cetera, all stocked up when you get there.

Road Trips

Bring Entertainment

You will need to have different items in your car to keep your twins entertained, nourished, and comfortable at each stage of their lives. For newborns, you'll need to make sure that you have plenty of diapers, wipes, formula/bottles, et cetera. As your twins get older, you'll need to pack things like DVDs, CDs, games, toys, snacks, sippy cups, and so much more. Consider the early times the easy times when it comes to car travel. Road travel with infants is actually a lot easier than it sounds. Keep in mind that the younger the children, the more likely they are to sleep in the car. The rhythm of the road always lulls me right to sleep (when I'm not driving, of course), and it will do the same thing to your babies.

Oh, Sheet

If you're planning on making a lot of pit stops throughout your journey, bring a large bedsheet from home to throw over the picnic table, to place on the grass, or to put anywhere that your babies might get to have some tummy or crawling time. Don't bring your finest linens for this; a simple bedsheet will go a long way. Just decide ahead of time which side is going to be facedown so that you can use the "correct" side every time.

Take It Mile by Mile

If you're taking an extended road trip, make sure that you leave plenty of time for rest stops. You should try to keep your babies on the same schedule that they were on at home. This means if you were feeding them every three hours, you need to make sure that you stop every three hours to feed them on your trip. Planning ahead will help you plan your route better. If you'll be traveling mostly on highways, you may want to get off the highway and settle into a nice small town ahead of feeding time instead of having to frantically feed them at a rest stop.

Hotels

A Room for Two (or More)

Before you book your hotel stay, inquire about what supplies they have that might help make your load a little lighter. Do they have Pack 'n Plays or minicribs? Some hotels even have full-size cribs available. It will also be helpful to know if there is a refrigerator in the room so that you can plan out how you will handle feedings on your trip. If you can, get a room with a kitchenette so that you can avoid having every meal in a restaurant. Don't trust the hotel website for the latest information. Sometimes hotel chains that are run by large corporations have particular items "standard" in a room but aren't always actually in the room. Call the hotel that you're booking directly to make sure that the items you're looking for are really there, in working order, and that you can use them during your stay. It would stink to find out that a family who checked in ten minutes before you got the last crib in the hotel.

Also think about how big of a room you will need. If it's just you, your spouse, and your twins, a room with two double beds should have more than enough space, but check before you book it. Maybe a room with a king-size bed actually has more square footage than a room with two smaller beds. Your little ones will be sleeping in a crib or cribs anyway, so maybe getting one bigger bed will be your best bet. If you're traveling with additional children or family members, check and see if the hotel offers adjoining rooms. Sometimes, booking adjoining rooms is cheaper than booking a suite and might even offer more square footage. Again, call the hotel and get all of the details before making your decision.

Alternate Options

Broaden your horizons and look beyond the obvious hotels and motels when you're planning a trip. Sometimes condo developments, or even homes, open themselves up for short-term rentals. Websites like www.home exchange.com, www.homeaway.com, and www.airbnb.com must have been created with families of twins in mind.

Safety Kits

Any time you leave your own home, you also leave the safety of its surroundings. There are some great products on the market that make it really easy for you to baby-proof on the road. Safety is something that you should always have in the forefront of your mind, no matter where you're heading. There is a great product called Travel-Tot, which includes all the baby-proofing equipment you need for a hotel room. If you plan to travel a lot with your twins, add this item to your registry list!

Prepping for Your Surrogate's Delivery

Preparing for your twins' arrival via surrogate? Packing for the birth can be very overwhelming, but don't forget that they have diapers, wipes, formula, and all of the basics wherever it is that your babies will be delivered. If you are flying to your destination, it is important to prioritize. You can't bring the entire nursery with you. The suggestions from our Twiniversity families who had their twins via surrogate for what to bring are as follows:

- Bottles—washed and ready to go.
- A bottle brush and a drying rack to set up in the hotel room. We suggest bringing something simple and inexpensive, as you most likely won't travel home with it.
- Microwave steamer bags—these work great in hotel rooms.
- Infant car seats
- Swaddle blankets
- Newborn hats
- Onesies
- Sleepers
- Carriers/slings—these are perfect for traveling and bonding with your new little ones.

Twins Take Flight

Nothing can scare parents of twins more than the idea of flying with two babies. How will you manage? What will you bring? Will you survive the flight without being pelted by peanuts from the people in the neighboring rows? The good news is that flying with twins can be manageable if you follow my tried-and-true rules, retain a sense of humor, and don't forget to bribe your seatmates. Here are my best tips for flying with twins.

Getting Around the Airport

To make getting from point A to point B easier, you should think about how you are going to spend the time waiting at the airport. The first thing you should do is check the most recent federal guidelines for flying with your children. The most updated info can be found at www.DHS.gov/Trip. There you can find out what liquids you can take on the plane and if your children need to wear their shoes while going through security. These rules get updated regularly, so check them as your departure date gets closer. Many airports now even have a security lane just for families. Take advantage of this perk whenever possible. If you are planning on taking your car seats with you, you may also want to consider buying a special travel bag for them so they don't get too scuffed up when going through baggage check.

Traveling Around the Terminal

Once you arrive, think about how you want to get your children around the terminal. Stick to gate checking your stroller the first year, and make sure that your airline will accept your specific one. Rules change all the time and you don't want to have to get stuck bringing it all the way back to the front of the terminal or having to check it right when you get there.

If you are leaving the stroller at home, you have several travel options. A few companies make wheeled carts that attach to a convertible car seat, allowing it to act as a stroller. If this sounds like a good option to you, check with your local twins club about borrowing something like this. It may not be worth the investment if you travel once a year or less.

If you aren't bringing your car seats with you, think about how you are getting from the airport to the place you're staying on the other side. Some car rental companies will charge you an additional fee but can provide you with car seats. If that's your plan, be sure to reserve them ASAP. Rental companies usually have very limited supplies of car seats.

Don't Fly Too Soon

Most pediatricians recommend that you wait at least eight weeks before taking your twins on a flight. While some airlines will allow you to fly with younger infants, it's always best to follow your doctor's advice. If an infant under eight weeks old gets a cold, it can be a big problem, so evaluate the risk against how important this trip really is.

Pack Extra Extras

Did you know that most airports don't sell baby gear? Good luck trying to find a diaper, wipe, or even some formula after passing security. Make sure to bring much more than you need. One Twiniversity member arrived at her destination diaperless because she underestimated how many she would need. Don't let that happen to you!

Go Off-Season

If you aren't locked into particular dates, find out when the slow season is for your destination. Holidays are usually the busiest travel times of the year, so booking your flight for the week or two *after* major holidays will typically ensure that it will be a little less crowded where you are headed.

If you are traveling overseas, call the hotel and do your homework on when their slow season is. Of course, the weather might not be perfect, but with new twins, it's not a bad idea to avoid crowds, so this is the time to go. Another money saver is to travel on Tuesdays, when flights are cheapest.

Time It Right

If your twins are on a schedule, try to book your flights around their naps. If they typically nap at 11 a.m., try to be airborne at 10 a.m. so they have a moment to chill, take in their surroundings, and get ready for their nap. Also, the first flight of the day is always a good option, too, since it's almost always on time.

Pick the Right Seats

Federal guidelines allow babies to fly as "lap infants" (for free) until they are two years old. This means that if you are flying with your partner and the twins, you can each hold one of the twins throughout the flight and pay nothing extra for them. However, airplanes only have one extra oxygen mask per row. This means that if you're traveling with two adults and two babies, you cannot both sit with lap infants in the same row with three seats because there will only be an oxygen mask for one baby. Airlines should know this and should not book the seats this way, but it's important for you to know it, too, so that you don't book seats in two different rows and then switch to sit next to each other because that seat is empty or if the nice lady next to one of you would rather fly in steerage than sit next to someone with a lap infant.

That said, if you are sitting in a row of three seats and can possibly afford it, it's not a bad idea to pay for a third seat. With three seats, you don't have to worry about the oxygen mask thing. You can bring a car seat on the plane as a "home base" for one of the babies and play hot potato with the other. Just think, if one of you has to go to the bathroom, the other doesn't have to manage both babies because one can sit in that car seat in the third seat.

Once you decide how many seats you're buying, you have to decide where to sit on the plane. Most people think that the last row of the plane is the worst place to sit, and that's why it's the very best place when you're flying with twins. First of all, if you sit there with two babies, the flight attendants will (probably) take pity on you and bring you anything you need. Second, you can only annoy the people in front of you—there's nobody behind you to worry about.

As my kids got older, I found that if I sat in the back, I could go to the bathroom, keep the door open, and still see everybody. Seriously, I did this. Plus, the people in the back of the plane are just nicer. The people in front are the frequent travelers. They want to get on and get off as quickly as possible. The people in the back are often with children as well. Either way, they'll be more sympathetic. True, the seats in the back don't recline, but you're not going to be able to relax or take a nap anyway, so who cares?

When booking an international flight with twins, I strongly recommend that you find out if the airline has bulkhead seats with infant bassinets. If this is the case, as it often is, make sure to plan your trip ahead of time so that you can book those seats. On international flights, lap infants are often free, but sometimes they charge 10 percent extra to book the seats with the bassinets. Call a service representative instead of booking online to make sure it's done correctly and you know exactly how much you will be charged. Also be aware that the bassinets on international flights are fairly shallow. Ask the airline for the dimensions to be sure your twins will fit! Don't plan on relying solely on those bassinets to contain your children. It's a good idea to also take a baby carrier on board with you so that your babies can have a home base when they're not in the bassinet.

Win Over Your Neighbors

Bring a handful of earplugs on board and pass them out to the people seated around you. You know that when they see you coming down the aisle with twins, they might be cursing you out under their breath, but the earplugs will definitely help you win them over. Whether they end up needing the earplugs or not, they will be on your side and that's really all that matters.

Have Your "Go Bag"

On the plane, you'll need to have a "go bag" for each child, containing diapers, wipes, and a change or two of clothes. This way, you can take one baby to the bathroom at a time for a quick change, even in the airport. When you go to the bathroom on the plane, just take what you need. Those bathrooms are small.

Pack for a Feeding Frenzy

You'll also want to bring enough formula and baby food for at least two more feeds than you think you'll need in the air. You never know how long you might get stuck on that tarmac. Baby food, breast milk, and formula are allowed through security; they will be hand inspected.

Breast-feeding in the Air

If you're breast-feeding, try to sit in the window seat to avoid capturing the attention of everyone who is on their way to or from the restroom. You might also want to bring a breast-feeding cover like Bebe au Lait. No, you shouldn't feel ashamed or like you have to cover up, but many babies over three months old will get distracted by all the commotion and have a hard time nursing otherwise. Remember to nurse during takeoff and landing if possible. The constant swallowing helps prevent the babies' ears from hurting as the pressure changes. If you can't fathom tandem feeding during takeoff (and who could blame you?), plan to nurse one baby and have your partner bottle-feed the other.

Change the Bottle Nipples

After your twins graduate from Level 1 bottle nipples, hold on to them for future plane rides. During takeoff and landing, feed your babies with Level 1 nipples because they require the babies to suck and swallow more, which helps them clear their ears. It's important for them to drink, not only because of the pressure, but also to keep them hydrated. Think about giving them a bottle of juice as a "treat" if your doctor says it's okay.

Reach Out Locally

No matter where you go in this world, when you get to your destination, find the local parents of a twins club. More often than not, if you contact a local parents-of-twins club before your trip, you won't have to bring or rent much baby gear because someone local will offer to lend it to you. You don't even have to bring a stroller. Someone might even meet you at the airport with everything you need. This is a courtesy that parents with twins often pass on to each other. We are an underground secret society that looks out for each other. If you connect, we'll help you.

CHAPTER 12

keeping the foundation strong, or "batman and chocolate milk"

F YOU ARE SIMPLY READING THIS CHAPTER IN SEQUENCE WITH THE REST of the book, I think that's a good sign. The fact that your spouse means enough to you to not skip over this part tells me that you value your relationship. That's a good start. If you've cracked this book open again after your twins are born and you and your spouse are going through a rough patch, that's an even better sign. Now you're dealing with the effects of sleep deprivation along with the stress of caring for twins, and you still value your marriage enough to work on it.

Twins can hit your marriage like a hurricane. If you fail to prepare yourselves, want things to improve immediately, and only see the damage, it can destroy you. But if you take the time to prepare correctly, have the patience to wait it out, and maintain the right attitude, it can actually be a fun and exciting adventure. I very often hear from parents of twins who are going through a trying time in their marriages, and this is no surprise. They struggle with money issues, stress, work, sex, lack of sex, feeling unappreciated, and more.

I've been through the storm with several of our Twiniversity couples.

I've heard both sides of the story, and have learned so much from our wise members. I'm no marriage expert, but I've been through this myself, too, and in this chapter I'll give you the best advice I could gather on keeping your marriage together (and happy) during your twins' first year.

Your Marriage Is a Priority

Close your eyes (well, read this first) and picture your future. Imagine yourself on a porch swing on a nice summer day with a cool glass of iced tea in your hand. Everything is calm and peaceful. Now look next to you. Is anyone sitting on that porch swing with you? I hope you are envisioning your spouse.

If you've been married for a while, you realize by now that marriage is work. I don't know one couple that was just handed a perfect marriage. All of the couples I know (that are still together) have had to put a lot of effort into making their marriage a success. I am sad to say that I have plenty of friends who have already been married and divorced just in the time since my twins were born. When I hear about yet another divorce, I just become very thankful for my partner in crime, John.

My husband always jokes about the fact that he never wanted to have kids and that I am the one who forced him into this whole thing. When I see him now playing with our twins, I think about how lucky he is that I coerced him into something that brings him so much joy, but I also think about how hard those early days of their lives were on our marriage. I don't think that John ever outright resented me for talking him into having kids, but the pressures from work, from me about wanting him at home more to help care for the babies, and from the twins themselves and all of their needs definitely added up.

It is these pressures and these stresses that can cause real damage to a marriage if you're not careful. I recently went to a twin parent gathering in New York City and ran into a couple that had previously attended my Twiniversity 101 class. It was so great to see them after their twins had arrived and were already six months old. After showing me some beautiful

From the MOM Squad: "*Don't blame each other when times get tough. Remain a team.*" —Megan F.

photos, the mom walked away and started talking with another parent. The dad said to me, "Nat, got a minute?" We sat down and he told me a story.

A few days before, the father had forgotten his keys at home when he went to work. At the end of the day, he returned home, where he knew that his wife, their nanny, and his twins were resting. He told me that he rang the doorbell for over an hour and was about to give up when his wife finally came to the door. When she opened it, she simply said, "You know, you aren't the priority anymore."

This gentleman is a mogul in the New York City business world, and he was breaking down before me. He explained how he knew that the kids were the priority now, but he didn't know he would be completely cast aside for them. The dad went on to say that he didn't know what more he could do. His wife had full-time help. He did whatever she asked. He rushed home each night to be with his family and was greeted with a dismissal instead of a welcome. I explained to this dad that the first year is rough and that it isn't uncommon for a dad to feel temporarily cast aside. But I knew that this situation was extreme. I reminded him that once the twins were sleeping through the night and he and his wife got some time alone, things would get better. His reply was, "If we make it that long."

My heart broke for him. It still does. It must have been hard for him to open up in the first place, but he seemed like he had already given up. Though things had only been bad for a few months, it seemed like it was already too late and I wish he had gotten help sooner. Never assume that a problem in your marriage is simply a bump in the road. Especially with the daily stress and challenges of twins in the house, a bump can quickly turn into a hill, a hill into a mountain, et cetera.

I'll be the first to tell you that every marriage goes through times like this. The important thing is to stop it before it goes too far and it becomes even more difficult (if not impossible) to get back to a loving partnership. The first few years of my twins' lives really tested my own marriage. My husband was my high school sweetheart and we've now been married for thirteen years, but at times I have wondered if I would be happier without him. I'm sure he has thought the same thing about me. But when it came down to it, I always knew that my kids would be the ones to lose out if I bailed. So with each "bump," I worked a little harder, and he did, too.

Never forget how important your marriage is to your kids. When your twins are born, you might look at them and think that they are the most important things in the world, but they're not. It may sound weird, but your marriage is actually more important. Do you know why? Because your marriage is the most important thing to *them*. Your marriage or partnership is what gives your kids a sense of safety and security. It will define for them what a marriage is.

Do you ever hear about friends or colleagues unwittingly repeating the mistakes in their parents' marriages? This is because our parents define marriage for all of us. We only know what we see firsthand at home, and what your twins see in your home will shape their view of marriage for their entire lives. It doesn't start later, when your twins are "old enough to understand," either. Babies pick up on everything—anger, yelling, fights, affection, and love. No matter how young your twins are, never forget that you are already the first role models in their lives. If you are a good, loving, faithful spouse, they will learn to be the same from watching you. That is why I call this chapter "Keeping the Foundation Strong." (You'll find out about the other half of the title in a bit.) Your marriage is truly the foundation for your twins' lives. Here are some of my top tips for keeping it rock solid.

Talk It Out

When was the last time that you and your spouse actually talked? When you get busy with the babies, you may not notice until you haven't had a discussion with your partner in four days. I'm not talking about checking in with each other about the diapers, the dishes, and the other chores—I'm asking when the last time was that you really talked? How does he feel about being a new father? How do you feel about being a new mother? Talk about things you used to talk about, not just the weather, or local news, or an upcoming election. Talk about something that really matters to you.

R-E-S-P-E-C-T

It sounds so obvious, but don't forget to treat each other with respect. Both of you play very important roles in your twins' lives. One is not more important than the other. I've watched so many families grow resentful of each other. The worker bee gets jealous of the person who gets to stay home with the babies, and the person at home with the babies feels resentful of the person who gets to get out of the house every day! Remember that you are a team, and that one part of your team will not work without the other.

Compliment Each Other

Whether it's a friend or a stranger on the street, it's always nice to get a compliment from someone. Why not take a moment to pay your spouse a compliment? It doesn't have to be about something superficial. Maybe they changed a diaper in record time or just invented a really cute game with the twins. Take notice. It's these little things in life that often get overlooked, and complimenting and encouraging each other will go a long way.

From the MOM Squad: *"You and your partner need to be a team. Don't let gender roles or one person working and the other at home get in the way of your teamwork. You will be happiest and sanest if you split the work as equally as possible." —Amanda A.*

Take Time

If you are in the middle of a heated argument, don't just storm out of the room or let yourself boil over and say things that you'll regret. Simply let your spouse know that you need a minute. Go in the other room and take a deep breath, or go for a walk to cool off. Chances are that you'll be able to calm down and speak to your partner more calmly when you return.

Love Means Always Saying "I'm Sorry"

Marriage is not a battle of wills. It doesn't really matter who's right and who's wrong, does it? Isn't it much more important to stay together and be happy? A simple "I'm sorry" goes so far in toning down an argument or even preventing a major blowout. Say it often and with sincerity!

Check In Daily

It's easy to become disconnected from your spouse with all of your new responsibilities, but don't forget the importance of a quick phone call in the middle of a busy day. Call or text just to say hi. Ask your spouse how their day is going. Don't forget that you are partners first and foremost, and checking in on each other is an important part of this partnership.

Take Time for You

It can be hard to feel loving and patient with your spouse if you are crazed from taking care of the babies all day and don't have a moment to hear yourself think. It may sound counterintuitive, but time for yourself will greatly improve your time at home. Don't just assume that you'll find some time for yourself at some point during the week. Schedule it in and encourage your partner to do the same.

Jump in with Both Feet

If you're holding on to past resentments or always looking to be right, your marriage will have a hard time withstanding the pressure of twins. Try to let go of all that and jump back into your marriage with the same commitment that you had in the beginning. Exchange new vows or make new promises to each other. It's important to remind each other why you're there! Let go of the past and commit yourself to making this work.

Don't Question Each Other

News flash—your husband is not going to do things the exact same way as you, and that is okay! When it was my husband's time to take care of the twins, they would pretend that they were doggies and he would have them crawling around eating Cheerios out of bowls on the floor. Was this my favorite mess to come home to? No. Did I tell him to stop playing this game? No. (But I wanted to.) As long as he is following the same basic house rules as you and nobody is in danger, let him do things his way. If you hover and instruct him every step of the way, he'll never figure it out for himself.

Get Out into the World

Date nights are an absolute must! Yes, babysitters can be costly, and so can restaurants and movies, but you need to find a way to make it happen. It is a very worthy investment for the future of your entire family. Forget going to fancy restaurants, and go on simple dates where you can talk and reconnect. It can be as easy as going for a long walk, a cocktail, or a game of darts. Just get out into the big world and remind each other what it's like to be out there with each other.

Make Marriage a Priority

Your marriage should be the most important thing in your life. If you have to make sacrifices in order to keep it on track, so be it. Not only is your marriage important, but so is your partner's happiness. Supporting him or her in their endeavors will only strengthen your partnership and keep you both on the right track.

Listen as Much as You Talk

Don't forget that your spouse is a separate person with his or her own feelings, opinions, hopes, dreams, and frustrations. It's important to tell your partner what you want and need, but it's equally essential that you listen to what he or she has to say, too. Keep an open mind and never assume that your needs are more important than his or hers.

Try Not to "Keep Score"

What's more important: being right or being happy? Put your ego aside and focus on the health of the marriage. Make decisions—big and small—based on this. Is it better for your marriage to apologize or to keep fighting? Is it better for your marriage to complain about how your spouse always leaves a towel on the bathroom floor or to just let it go? Here's another way of thinking about it—if your marriage falls apart, then nobody wins, especially your twins, so there is no such thing as a "winner" and a "loser" if you do everything you can to make it work.

Remember Why You Got Married in the First Place

Do you remember those traits that made you fall in love with your spouse to begin with? Was it his sense of humor, integrity, or intelligence? Was it simply those baby blue eyes? Take some time to think about why you chose this person to share your life with and then try to keep appreciating those traits all these years later.

Be the Person You Want Your Children to Marry

Sure, it's too early to think about what kind of girl little Matteo is going to bring home, but it's never too early to be that girl. No, I'm not going Freudian on you. Your marriage is simply the model that your children will most likely follow when it's their turn to get married one day. Your kids trust you implicitly and will assume (unless taught otherwise) that you are behaving the way that married people are meant to behave. So go ahead and be the person that you want your kids to marry and the person that you want your kids to be in their own marriages one day.

> **Note from Dad:**   "Most of our focus has been directed toward our boys since they were born, so it's strained our relationship. It's getting better as the boys get older, because my wife and I find more time for just us. It's important to tend to your partner as much as your twins because at the end of the day, you all need each other." —*Timothy G.*

Remember That Porch Swing

You need to work to make sure that your marriage stays intact. Everybody worries about preparing their bodies for the delivery of their twins and preparing their homes for the arrival of their newborns. Not many people think about how their marriage is going to withstand the impact of this monumental life event. Take notice now, and see what you can do to make sure that you stay in touch with the love of your life. Having children will actually make your bond stronger if you work hard, take notice, and pay attention to each other.

Sex after Twins

It's so common for your sex life to take a major backseat after twins are born. Singleton parents go through this, too! After the birth, your hormones are telling you not to have sex because your body doesn't want to get pregnant again. (This is especially true if you're nursing.) It's hard to trick Mother Nature and find that desire for sex despite this. Plus, you're sleep deprived, haven't showered in days, can't remember the last time you ate food off a plate, and certainly can't imagine how to find time for sex with two babies to take care of.

I will be very honest here and tell you that I actually made the opposite mistake and got back in the saddle too soon after my twins were born. My kids were only home from the NICU for a few days before we made a go of it. I wasn't so interested in the sex itself, but I craved that feeling of closeness and normalcy after everything that we had been through. Sorry if this is TMI, but it was bad. My body was just not ready, and it was painful and awkward, and (for no logical reason) I secretly blamed my husband. That didn't exactly do wonders for our relationship, but we worked through it.

Most doctors will suggest that you wait at least six weeks after the birth before bringing sexy back, and I hope that my story has taught you to listen to your doctor! Make sure that you are healed and healthy enough to enjoy lovemaking when you do get back to it, but don't use this as an excuse to put it off forever, either. Talk to your spouse about your sex life and be honest about your reasons for not feeling ready. Don't just ignore it and let it become the elephant in the room.

You might need to make adjustments to your love life now that the twins are here. Well, you've had to make adjustments to every other part of your life, so this should come as no surprise, right? If you're too tired to have sex at night, try having sex in the afternoon—what's so bad about that? When our twins were little, we never had a moment to ourselves because there was always at least one baby awake or a family member around. It was always something. We had to be resourceful and find a way to fit it in. Don't forget that this can be fun and really revitalize your sex life if you keep the right attitude!

Eventually, John and I got creative and came up with a plan that really worked for us. It was called "Batman and chocolate milk." When the twins were old enough to watch TV and mature enough to be left unattended for a few minutes, they loved watching *Batman* cartoons and it was a real treat for them. If it had been a while and the mood struck one of us, John or I would look at the other and say, "Batman and chocolate milk?" We'd make them a small cup of chocolate milk, put on an episode of *Batman*, close the door, and get down to business. This did wonders for our marriage, so never forget that there is a light at the end of the tunnel. It might just take a little creativity and patience in order to find it. Just be sure your twins are old enough for Batman and chocolate milk before you steal a few moments alone.

conclusion

YOU DID IT! WHETHER YOUR TWINS HAVE TURNED ONE OR YOU'VE SIMPLY finished reading this book, take a moment to congratulate yourself on reaching an important milestone.

It seems like just yesterday that my twins took their first steps. It was a minute ago that they said their first words. It was a second ago that I heard them say, "I love you, Mommy" for the first time. Time flies by so fast, so make sure to cherish each moment as it comes. Never let the stress become more important than the precious babies right in front of you. If I could give you one last piece of advice, it would be this—take lots of pictures and make sure to back them up! We have lost two computers since our twins were born and lost all of the photos on the hard drive along with them.

Never forget that every day is an opportunity to create memories, and a new chance to raise your children the way that you want them to be raised. No matter how hard yesterday was, you'll have the gift of a new day with every sunrise. There is no more important or difficult job in life than being a parent. There's no sick time, no paid vacation days, and not even overtime, but you can't beat the bonuses. My twins are my reasons for living. They make me want to be a better person every day because they think the best of me even when I don't think it of myself.

The road ahead of you will be long and occasionally bumpy, but the good news is that you are not alone. By having twins, you are not only guaranteed a playmate for your children, but also a built-in support network for yourself that is unlike any other in the world. I will be here for you whenever you need me, and don't forget that any questions, fears, or concerns that may be keeping you up at night have probably been asked before. Our twin parent community is one of the strongest in the world, and you have all of the answers at your fingertips on our Twiniversity.com forums and website. Good luck and enjoy!

XXOO,
Nat

acknowledgments

I'VE BEEN VERY FORTUNATE IN MY LIFE TO BE SURROUNDED BY SUCH amazing, inspiring, and dedicated folks who want the best and more for me. It's because of them that this book was even *remotely* possible. My family, my friends, and my twin parenting community deserve an enormous thank-you for their unwavering support. So, I tip my hat to you all! Thank you so much for making my dream come true—not only with these pages, but for allowing Twiniversity to become a world-recognized online community exclusively for us!

There are a few people who deserve an extra bit of thanks. Here they are:

I'd like to thank Lucia Watson, my editor at Penguin and fellow twin mom. You, above all, understand the importance of this book and I wish that I wrote it earlier just for you. Thanks, too, to the entire team at Avery for turning this book into a reality.

I'd like to thank J. L. Stermer, Paul Fedorko, and the entire N. S. Beinstock gang for getting me exactly where I wanted to be.

I'd like to thank Judith Regan, who saw something more in my idea than anyone else and taught me how dreaming big isn't big enough. You can always dream bigger. I did dream bigger thanks to her.

I'd like to thank Diane Reverand, who started this project with me and gave it the chops to grow into what it is today.

I'd also like to thank Siri, yes, *that* Siri. I've always considered myself more of a public speaker than a writer, and Siri has made the transition smooth as silk. A very good portion of this book was "spoken" as opposed to written thanks to Siri. So a big thank-you to the folks at Apple for making this public speaker an author.

I'd like to thank the love of my life, John, for being so patient and understanding. I know that we always joke that we are the worst gift givers, but I think we both scored big with the Diaz Duo! Thank you for the best gift of all.

I'd like to thank my sister, Viv (aka "Sis"), who is my biggest fan, my best friend, my No. 1 babysitter, and a big reason why I never give up. This one is for you!

I'd like to thank my parents, Camille and Eddie, who showed me what true love is and set the bar for what a good parent is supposed to be.

I'd like to thank my aunt Viv, aka Auntie, for buying the twins breakfast *every* Saturday morning so I could either get a few pages written or a few more minutes of sleep. You also taught me how to be a tough cookie—thanks for that one!

I'd like to thank my in-laws, Francine and Roger, for supporting the crazy life I live. Yes, it's hectic, but you guys help me keep it together.

I'd like to thank other members of my family, including Aunt Mandy, Uncle Allie, Mike, Grandma Julie, the Mulraneys, and the rest of my amazing bunch who make living in a pack the best experience a person can have. There is no way I could have done this (book or having twins) without all of you.

I'd like to thank Dr. Ana Barbieri, my obstetrician. Dr. Barbieri, if it weren't for you, my fingers would not be touching this keyboard. I credit my life to you and hope you see I'm putting it to good use.

I'd like to thank Dr. Marie Keith and the entire staff of Soho Pediatrics for supporting my family in all those sickly dark hours.

I'd like to thank Liz, my nurse in the Mount Sinai NICU. You have no idea how much you helped me in my darkest hours. You were our nurse and our friend. You became part of our family. A hundred thanks to you.

I'd like to thank my Twiniversity Mom Squad: Talitha, Jill, Sarah, Frankie, and the rest of the gang who always saw what Twiniversity was meant to be and helped it (and continue to help it) grow.

I'd like to thank my Pro Mom Squad: Traci Zeller, Ann Gugle, Annie Bradley, Joan Friedman, Dr. Barbara Deli, Shari Bayles, and Dr. Preeti Parikh. I'd also like to thank Asaf R. for his two cents on being a dad-only family and Laurie H. on being a mom-only family.

A *very* special thank-you to Sara Willhite, Twiniversity member who also helped name this book after struggling with the title for ages! *Thank you, Sara!*

I'd like to thank my friends Melissa, Valentina, Miriam, and the rest of my peeps who always gave me feedback when I had an idea or even just an ear to listen to me vent.

I'd like to thank all the twin moms who have inspired me: Mary Grace Roach, Mary Elizabeth Brennan, Tara Telford, Cassandra Bolz, and the many others who have shared their lives with me. I'm a better mom, and a better person, because I know you.

I'd like to thank *all* the members of the Manhattan Twins Club for giving me the support I needed when I first found out the big news *and* for still supporting me to this day.

I'd like to thank Jodi Lipper, the best writer a gal could ever have. You know better than anyone else that there is no way I could have done this without you. You are a tough cookie and I'm glad you are on my side. You took my words, thoughts, and ideas and transformed them into these pages that you have in your hands. You kept me on track and made me keep my deadlines when I never thought I would. Thank you for your patience, kindness, and encouragement. Thank you for your hard work and dedication. I'm proud of our partnership. Now let's get another mani/pedi while the kids are in school!

Above all else, I would like to thank my twins, Anna and John. I had no idea what I was getting into when you were born. I'm happy to say that every sleepless night, every moment from then till now was all worth it.

Anna, you're the funniest person I know. No matter what anyone tells you in life, just be yourself and you will move mountains. You are my No. 1 girl in the whole wide world.

Johnny, I've never met a kid more generous and caring than you. You make me want to be a better person every day of my life. You are my No. 1 boy in the whole wide world.

You are both the most amazing people I know. I am proud of the two of you every day. When you grow up, and read this, know that I love you more than all the stars in the sky and all of the fish in the sea. I thank God every day that you were chosen to be my babies. I love you both.—Mommy

appendix a
Birth Plan Checklist

Attendants and Amenities

I'd like the following people to be present during labor and/or birth:

☐ *Partner:* _____

☐ *Friend/s:* _____

☐ *Relative/s:* _____

☐ *Doula:* _____

☐ *Children:* _____

I'd also like:

☐ *To bring music*

☐ *To dim the lights*

☐ *To wear my own clothes during labor and delivery*

☐ *To take pictures and/or film during labor and delivery*

Pain Relief

I'd like to try the following pain-management techniques:

☐ *Acupressure*

☐ *Bath/shower*

☐ *Breathing techniques/distraction*

☐ *Hot/cold therapy*

☐ *Self-hypnosis*

☐ *Massage*

☐ *Medication*

☐ *Please don't offer me pain medication. I'll request it if I need it.*

If I decide I want medicinal pain relief, I'd prefer:

☐ *Regional analgesia (an epidural and/or spinal block)*

☐ *Systemic medication*

Labor

- [ ] *I'd like the option of returning home if I'm not in active labor.*

Once I'm admitted, I'd like:

- [ ] *My partner to be allowed to stay with me at all times*
- [ ] *Only my practitioner, nurse, and guests present (i.e., no residents or medical students)*
- [ ] *To wear my contact lenses, as long as I don't need a C-section*
- [ ] *To eat if I wish to*
- [ ] *To stay hydrated by drinking clear fluids instead of having an IV*
- [ ] *To walk and move around as I choose*

As long as the babies and I are doing fine, I'd like:

- [ ] *To have intermittent rather than continuous electronic fetal monitoring*
- [ ] *To be allowed to progress free of stringent time limits*

I plan to:

- [ ] *Breast-feed exclusively*
- [ ] *Combine breast-feeding and formula-feeding*
- [ ] *Formula-feed exclusively*

The following can be offered to my babies:

- [ ] *Formula*
- [ ] *Sugar water*
- [ ] *Pacifier*
- [ ] *Please don't offer anything to my twins at any point without my or my spouse's permission.*

I'd like my twins fed:

- [ ] *On demand*
- [ ] *On a schedule*

I'd like:

- [ ] *24-hour rooming-in with my babies*
- [ ] *My twins rooming-in with me only when I'm awake*

- [ ] *My babies brought to me for feedings only*
- [ ] *To make my decision later depending on how I'm feeling*

If one or both of my babies are male:

- [ ] *I'd like him (them) circumcised at the hospital*
- [ ] *I'll have him (them) circumcised later*
- [ ] *I don't want him (them) circumcised*

C-Section

If I have a C-section, I'd like:

- [ ] *My partner present at all times during the operation*
- [ ] *The screen lowered a bit so I can see my babies the moment they are born*
- [ ] *The babies given to my partner as soon as they're dried (as long as they are in good health)*
- [ ] *To breast-feed my babies in the recovery room*

Vaginal Birth

If they are available, I'd like to try:

- [ ] *A birthing stool*
- [ ] *A squatting bar*
- [ ] *A birthing chair*
- [ ] *A birthing pool/tub*
- [ ] *Do so instinctively*
- [ ] *Be coached on when to push and for how long*

I'd like to try the following positions for pushing (and birth):

- [ ] *Semi-reclining*
- [ ] *Side-lying position*
- [ ] *Squatting*
- [ ] *Hands and knees*
- [ ] *Whatever feels right at the time*
- [ ] *As long as my babies and I are doing fine, I'd like the pushing stage to be allowed to progress free of stringent time limits*

I'd like:

- ☐ To watch my babies being born using a mirror if possible
- ☐ To touch my children's heads as they crown
- ☐ The room to be as quiet as possible
- ☐ If possible, I'd like to play the following music _____
- ☐ To avoid an episiotomy at all costs
- ☐ My partner to help deliver our babies

After birth, I'd like:

- ☐ To hold my babies right away, putting off any procedures that aren't urgent
- ☐ To breast-feed as soon as possible
- ☐ To wait until the umbilical cord stops pulsating before it's clamped and cut
- ☐ My partner to cut the umbilical cord

Postpartum

After delivery, I'd like:

- ☐ All newborn procedures to take place in my presence
- ☐ My partner to stay with the babies at all times if I can't be there
- ☐ To stay in a private room
- ☐ To wait for a bed by a window, if no private room is available
- ☐ To have a cot provided for my partner

appendix b

Twins Daily Log

This is the bible when it comes to keeping track of your day. Make many copies!

Time	Baby A oz/min	Baby B oz/min	Notes A (mood, l/r boob, meds)	Notes B (mood, l/r boob, meds)	Pee A	Pee B	Poop A	Poop B

www.Twiniversity.com   Classes@Twiniversity.com

resources

··

THE BOOK MAY BE NEARING THE END, BUT THAT DOESN'T MEAN THAT I'M
done with you. For the next "chapter" of your twins' lives, we welcome you
to join us on our thriving online community at Twiniversity.com, where
you can connect to thousands of other twin families from around the
globe. We have busy online chat forums and thousands of articles written
just for parents like you.

Here are some additional resources that may be helpful, but you will
find a full and updated list at Twiniversity.com.

Bed Rest Support
Sidelines—High Risk Pregnancy Support Network
Sidelines.org

Breast-Feeding Guidance
La Leche League: The world leader in breast-feeding support. 800-
LALECHE (525-3243)
http://www.lalecheleague.org/

Similac: This resource has a 24/7 hotline to answer all your breast-feeding questions. 1-800-232-7677
https://similac.com/

High Order Multiples
MOST: Mothers of Supertwins: http://www.mostonline.org/

Loss of a Multiple/Bereavement:
The vast majority of the time, expectant families will welcome their new babies without any complications. However, the extra excitement that comes with expecting twins also brings an added risk of complications and some families may even lose one or both of the babies before or after the birth. Whether a high-risk situation is identified early in the pregnancy or the loss is sudden and unexpected, the grief of losing one or two babies is shattering.

If this happens to you, and I hope from the bottom of my heart that it does not, remember that you are not alone. Sadly, far too many families have experienced this before you. These websites can provide support, and you may wish to seek professional counseling or group counseling:
Twinless Twins: http://www.twinlesstwins.org/
Center for Loss in Multiple Births: http://www.climb-support.org/

Twin-to-Twin Transfusion Syndrome
Fetal Health Foundation: http://www.fetalhealthfoundation.org
TTTS Foundation: http://www.tttsfoundation.org/

Preemie Support
Graham's Foundation: http://www.grahamsfoundation.com
March of Dimes: http://www.marchofdimes.com

Cord Blood Banking
Cord Blood Registry: http://www.cordblood.com

Postpartum Depression
Postpartum Progress: http://postpartumprogress.org/
Postpartum Support International: http://www.postpartum.net/

Car Seat Safety
The Car Seat Lady: http://www.thecarseatlady.com/
National Highway Traffic Safety Administration: http://www.nhtsa.gov/

Strollers mentioned in this book
Baby Jogger: http://www.BabyJogger.com
Baby Trend: http://www.BabyTrend.com
Britax: http://www.Britax.com
Bumbleride: http://www.Bumbleride.com
Joovy: http://www.Joovy.com
StrollAir: http://www.StrollAir.com
Valco: http://www.Valco.com

Other companies mentioned in this book
Baby Proofing
International Association for Child Safety: http://www.iafcs.org
Munchkin: http://www.munchkin.com
Safety 1st: http://safety1st.djgusa.com
Travel-Tot: http://www.Travel-tot.com

Pacifiers
MAM: http://www.mambaby.com

Bottles
Dr. Brown's: http://www.drbrownsbaby.com

Breast-Feeding Covers
Bebe au Lait: http://www.bebeaulait.com

index